Cancer Rehabilitation

PATRICIA A. DOWNIE

Trained at St. Thomas' Hospital, London, and after junior posts has been successively Superintendent Physiotherapist, The Royal Marsden Hospital, London; Rehabilitation Officer, The Marie Curie Memorial Foundation, London; Superintendent Physiotherapist, The London Chest Hospital. Awarded a Fellowship of the Chartered Society of Physiotherapy 1975; a Winston Churchill Fellow 1976. Currently Nursing and Medical Editor, Faber and Faber London.

Cancer Rehabilitation
An Introduction for Physiotherapists
and the Allied Professions

PATRICIA A. DOWNIE, FCSP
A Winston Churchill Fellow, 1976

with a Foreword by
Professor ERIC WILKES, OBE, MA, FRCP, FRCGP,
 MRCPsych, DObstRCOG
*Professor of Community Care and General Practice,
Department of Community Medicine,
University of Sheffield Medical School*

FABER AND FABER
3 Queen Square
London

*First published in 1978
by Faber and Faber Limited
Printed in Great Britain by
Latimer Trend & Company Ltd, Plymouth
All rights reserved*

© *Patricia A. Downie, 1978*

CONDITIONS OF SALE
This book is sold subject to the condition that it shall not, by way of trade or otherwise, be lent, re-sold, hired out or otherwise circulated without the publisher's prior consent in any form of binding or cover other than that in which it is published and without a similar condition including this condition being imposed on the subsequent purchaser

---

British Library Cataloguing in Publication Data

Downie, Patricia A
    Cancer rehabilitation.
    1. Cancer patients—Rehabilitation 2. Physical therapy
    I. Title
    362.1'9'6994   RC262

ISBN 0-571-11162-9
ISBN 0-571-11163-7   Pbk

Tribulation worketh patience;
and patience, experience;
and experience, hope.

Romans V, 4-5

Contents

Illustrations	page 9
Foreword by Professor Eric Wilkes	11
Preface	15
Acknowledgements	19
1. A general background to cancer	21
2. A general outline of diagnostic methods	30
3. An outline of medical and surgical treatments	36
4. The philosophy of rehabilitation for cancer patients	46
5. The role of physiotherapy in the treatment of patients receiving chemotherapy	56
6. The role of physiotherapy in the treatment of patients receiving radiotherapy	66
7. Rehabilitation for patients with breast cancer	80
8. Rehabilitation for patients undergoing head and neck surgery	96
9. The role of physiotherapy in the treatment of patients undergoing surgery for miscellaneous conditions	111
10. Precautions to be understood, undertaken or observed by physiotherapists when treating patients with cancer	130
11. The place of physiotherapy in the care of the terminally ill and those with pain problems	136
12. The role of the physiotherapist in public education concerning cancer	147

13. **Nutrition and the rehabilitation of the cancer patient** by J. W. T. Dickerson, Ph.D.(Cantab.), F.I.Biol., Professor of Human Nutrition, University of Surrey and Jackie Tredger, B.Sc. (Surrey), S.R.D., Lecturer in Dietetics, University of Surrey ... 152

14. **The psychological impact of cancer** by G. P. Maguire, Senior Lecturer in Psychiatry, The University Hospital of South Manchester ... 172

Glossary ... 189

References ... 192

Bibliography ... 195

Useful organizations ... 197

Homes and hospices ... 198

Useful addresses of cancer organizations and special homes in the United States of America and Canada ... 200

Index ... 202

Illustrations

FIGURE

1. The 'hold' to support a thoracotomy incision with the patient in side-lying *page* 127

PLATES (between pages 112 and 113)
1. A normal xeroradiograph of the breast
2. A xeroradiograph showing a cancer of the breast
3. A normal lymphogram of the lower limbs
4. A lymphogram showing the filling defects in the inguinal and para-aortic nodes of a patient with follicular lymphoma
5. A patient kneels at the altar rail following right hip disarticulation and fitting of a tilting-table prosthesis
6. A paraplegic, Mr. S., standing initially, 3 months after becoming paralysed
7. Mr. S.'s progression to crutches
8. Mr. S. driving his automatic car
9. Mr. S. walking across the school playground
10. Mr. T. on admission with a total right hemiplegia from metastases in the frontal lobes
11. Mr. T. walking out of the department on the day of his discharge
12. Antero-lateral view of patient following Halsted radical mastectomy
13. The same patient with her prosthesis in position

14. The Jobst compression unit with the sleeve
15. A patient lying on a plinth receiving treatment with the Jobst compression unit
16. A lymphoedematous arm before treatment with the Jobst compression unit
17. The same arm after treatment
18. A female patient who has undergone hemi-mandibulectomy and removal of part of the floor of mouth with repair from a forehead graft
19. The same patient 12 months later
20. Physiotherapist and nurse combine to treat a patient's chest following laryngectomy

Foreword

One can trace three main areas of interest in the professional development of the physiotherapist over the last quarter of a century, and these have each in turn first dominated and then shrunk to a subordinate, but still persistent and worthwhile, activity.

First, the physiotherapist was encumbered with equal parts of enthusiasm and gadgetry and spent a good deal of time and effort in ameliorating, predictably with a variable success, chronic or acute rheumatic, traumatic, or vascular problems that were not life-threatening in themselves but what they lacked in menace they made up in associated disability, pain or inconvenience. Peripheral nerve injuries and intermittent claudication, frozen shoulder or the injured knee were typical examples of this period.

Then as anaesthetic techniques improved, surgical audacity and medical curiosity moved into more heroic operative or resuscitative adventures: and into this era of intensive care, at the right hand of anaesthetist, cardiologist, orthopaedic, neuro- or cardio-thoracic surgeon, came the physiotherapist, as a colleague vital to the recovery and rehabilitation of patients who previously could have been treated only by a cautious and defeatist conservatism.

Now, in an era of economic stringency and escalating medical costs, one sees that high-quality long-term supportive care has not been provided for the serious chronic disabilities of an ageing society: and it is to this area that the physiotherapist more and more is beginning to turn her attention.

The profession has developed specialist interests for the spinal injury, for example, or for the hemiplegic. It is likely that the greatest contribution of the physiotherapist to the backstrain or the stroke remain to be made, and that the number of working days lost with the former or the rather patchy rehabilitation of the latter will improve only slowly over the next decade.

The enthusiasm, the competence, and the imaginative and flexible approach of the physiotherapist, however, give one good grounds for confidence even in an age of shrinking resources. They allow us to see the approach of ever greater responsibility to, and co-operation with, the physiotherapist as a professional among equals. She will be not only on the wards but in the patient's home, she will be a central skill in the growing number of day units, she will request or arrange admission to in-patient care, she will be an educator of patient, relative and health care colleagues.

Perhaps most important of all she will be conscious of her rehabilitative triumphs not just as objectives gained but as states to be maintained as fully as possible for as long as possible. Her interests in the maintenance of independence, in the activities of daily living, in the quality of the patient's life, and of the family as the unit of care, stretch out into chronic locomotor and neurological disorders or the supervisory follow-up of the severe stroke, the difficult rheumatoid, the multiple sclerosis or the elderly fractured femur. To achieve this she will be relentlessly patient-centred, neither trapped in the parochial problems of the group practice nor totally restricted to the specialist hospital-based department.

One forecasts therefore a bright future for the physiotherapist: and in this monograph one can see already fully developed and in operation the skills, enthusiasms and attitudes one had been hoping for tomorrow or the day after. This book is to some degree therefore both a description and a prophecy.

It is a description of some twenty years of expert specialization in the rehabilitation of the patient with malignant disease. We see the variety, the unpredictability and the gravity of this group of diseases, and the tremendous value of physiotherapy not only pre- and post-operatively but also for patients with a short life-expectancy. Again and again the case histories show that there can be many exquisite triumphs short of cure. The paraplegic from a disseminated primary growth in the breast, the brain-damaged patient, the patient with multiple skeletal metastases, the deformities of the facial or pharyngeal tumours, all these problems and how they were tackled are vividly and heart-warmingly presented.

Professional barriers are quietly broken down and a multi-disciplinary team forged in a way that cannot have been easy even in a specialist research unit. The various modalities of treatment are described and a general background given that is more than adequate for its purpose.

And at the heart of the book is the message that the aim of the physiotherapist, and hopefully indeed of all health workers, is to keep the patient going, to give zest and life and achievement until oblivion takes over; and to do this neither with premature surrender nor with over-optimistic ambitions, by skill and experience married to a total professional commitment.

It is an impressive testament that will help to alter and create the very future that it foreshadows.

ERIC WILKES
Sheffield, 1976

Preface

The greater part of this book was originally offered as a dissertation, for which a Fellowship of the Chartered Society of Physiotherapy was awarded.

The seeds of this book were sown twenty-five years ago when, as a newly qualified physiotherapist, I saw a patient who was paralysed from the waist downwards due to a metastatic deposit from a primary breast tumour. She was treated with radiotherapy, recovered full use of her legs, and continued to live and lead a full life. This was a new concept to one who had been taught that paraplegics seldom, if ever, recovered muscle power, and that cancer was a disease to be feared.

This work is not intended to be a textbook, but a practical introduction to the whole problem of rehabilitative care for patients with a cancerous disease. I have tried to present it in a positive and objective manner without minimizing in any way the accepted seriousness of many forms of cancer. This is a field of work where 'quality of life', however short, is so much more important than extended survival at any price, and this is why physiotherapists and others should be prepared to go to great lengths to enable some patients to become independent, even if only for a short time.

I have sought to show how the physiotherapist can exercise all her skills and techniques, her adaptability and her ingenuity, and not least her willingness to co-operate with colleagues of other professions. This is work which can be richly rewarding as well as utterly frustrating, and the care and treatment of the patient with cancer must always be seen within the whole pattern of life, so that aims looked for and the goals achieved may be kept in perspective.

Cancer is not a disease in itself; it is a generic term used to describe a number of diseases including the leukaemias, brain tumours, breast tumours, melanoma, sarcoma and rodent ulcers. In turn many of these may be sub-divided into differing types, but for simplicity it is proposed to use the word cancer or malignant disease throughout this book, though it would be more precise to talk about the cancerous diseases. Indeed, there is now a school of thought who suggest that we should talk about the oncological diseases (Raven, 1973). Oncology is the modern science of study of the tumour (from the Greek *oncos*, a mass of tumour, and *logos*, to study). Overnight one cannot alter terminology or its implied meanings; far better to keep the traditional words but aim to change man's approach to them.

Cancer is as old as history itself, but unhappily there has always been attached to it the implied stigma that death was an inevitable consequence. This has led to the awful pessimism which still surrounds the disease today, as well as the familiar comment, 'He (or she) has cancer and there's nothing to be done,' or, what is almost worse, 'He (or she) has cancer, so why bother to give any active treatment.' This book is designed to give the lie to these statements, and the case-histories are eloquent testimonies of a positive philosophy.

In order that physiotherapists may apply their skills and techniques to help the patient, it is essential that they appreciate the basic facts of the disease and the general medical treatments which may be carried out. For this reason an outline of these aspects is included. It is of necessity brief, and I would recommend physiotherapists who may be working in hospitals and units which specialize in cancer care, to dip into textbooks and continually to broaden their background. No knowledge is ever wasted, and I would apply the words of St. Augustine in his *Confessions*, 'Tolle lege, tolle lege' (pick it up and read) very literally where the acquiring of background knowledge is concerned. Patients ask all kinds of questions, and it helps the establishment of good relationships if one can help them understand their condition in a simple manner.

Florence Nightingale laid down precepts and principles when she founded her School of Nursing at St. Thomas' Hospital. They have stood the test of time, and one of them states, 'Every patient shall be an honoured guest.' Let us remember that this embraces everything necessary for total patient care and understanding, and nowhere is this more required than in rehabilitation for the patient with cancer.

P. A. DOWNIE
September 1977

Acknowledgements

The writing of this book has only been possible through the help of many people, but it is right to thank first and foremost all the patients whom I have known and treated, and who by their forebearance, courage and determination to live their lives despite the diagnosis, have contributed so much to this work.

I acknowledge the unstinted help I have received from many colleagues at the Royal Marsden Hospital, London and Surrey, and particularly from the Photographic Department who have provided the photographs, and from the Diagnostic X-ray Department who provided the X-rays.

I am grateful to Professor Eric Wilkes, Professor of Community Care and General Practice, University of Sheffield, for kindly writing the Foreword; he has been a staunch friend and trusted adviser for many years. To Professor John Dickerson and Dr. Peter Maguire my thanks for writing the additional chapters and by so doing highlighting two essential facets necessary to total rehabilitation.

I thank the many physicians, surgeons and radiotherapists who in different hospitals over the last twenty-five years have taught me so much and who have entrusted their patients to my care, and I am grateful for permission to quote case-histories. I am particularly grateful to Mr. Ronald Raven, O.B.E., O.St.J., T.D., F.R.C.S. for sustained support and encouragement over many years; his enthusiasm and prophetic foresight has enabled great strides to be taken in this field of rehabilitation.

I am appreciative of the kindness of the widow and family of the patient in Plates 6, 7, 8 and 9 in allowing the face to be shown unmasked.

I thank all my physiotherapy colleagues who have suffered my idiosyncarcies and particularly my thanks to Miss Diana Gaskell, M.C.S.P., who read and constructively criticized the original dissertation.

Chapter 11 on terminal care owes much to the distinguished work and teaching of the late Sister Nagdalen S.S.M., Sister Superior at the Hostel of God, London. Lux perpetua luceat ei.

Faber & Faber Ltd. have been most patient! Miss Jean Cunningham has offered much kindly advice and Miss Heather Potter nobly typed the script as well as guiding me along the right lines—to both I offer sincere thanks. My thanks also to Audrey Besterman for Figure 1.

Finally, I record my thanks to my teaching hospital, St. Thomas' Hospital, London, and particularly to all those Nightingales who wittingly or unwittingly taught me so much more than physiotherapy.

The statement on Euthanasia from His Eminence, the late Cardinal John Heenan, is reproduced from *The Hour of Our Death*, by kind permission of the joint authors, Sylvia Lack and Richard Lamerton, and the publishers, Geoffrey Chapman Ltd.

The Editors of the *Nursing Mirror*, the *Nursing Times* and *Physiotherapy* have kindly allowed the use of pictures and material previously published in their papers.

William Heinemann Medical Books Ltd. as publishers and R. W. Raven as editor have allowed Plates 5, 6, 14, 16 and 17 to be reproduced from *Domiciliary Care for the Patient with Cancer*.

To all these publishers and authors I offer my thanks for their kind co-operation.

Chapter One: A general background to cancer

Historical background

The word 'cancer' is a latinised form of the Greek *carcinoma*, meaning a crab. It has been suggested that the medical usage may have been inspired by the large veins which often surround a malignant growth and which to ancient 'quacks' suggested the claws of a crab; indeed, Galen writes, 'As a crab is furnished with claws on both sides of the body, so, in this disease (? cancer of the breast), the veins which extend from the tumour represent with it a figure much like a crab'.

Paul of Aegina (A.D. 625) writes similarly, 'However, some say that cancer is so called because it adheres with such obstinacy to the part it seizes, that like the crab, it cannot be separated from it without great difficulty'.

In astronomy, Cancer represents the constellation lying between Leo and Gemini, and even today there is a rather surprising superstition that there is a connection between Cancer, the sign of the Zodiac, and cancer, the disease, and that those born under the sign are predestined to die of the disease. It is precisely these latter thoughts which should inspire all who work with cancer patients to speak out fearlessly and express the hopes and reassurances which can be the antidote to these fearful 'old wives' tales'. Over and over again one still meets these tales and they are so zealously believed that it is extremely difficult to dispel them.

Some of the earliest accounts of cancer can be found recorded on Egyptian papyrus scrolls, particularly the Edwin Smith Surgical

Papyrus and the Ebers Papyrus. Both record cases of sarcoma, of pharyngeal cancer and of breast cancer; many of the latter are recorded as being treated by cauterization with a fire drill. (Today the cautery is still used by Bedouin doctors, and the author vividly recalls cautery scars on the back of an Arab patient who had been treated unsuccessfully by this method. He had suffered acute pains in his back and was finally flown to England where cancer of the pancreas was diagnosed. Following palliative surgery his pains subsided.) In this use of cautery, physiotherapists will of course recognize the principle of counter-irritation, as can be performed with local doses of ultraviolet light.

Later we read in the writings of the Greek historian, Herodotus, that in 430 B.C. Atossa had a growth in her breast which was ulcerating and spreading. While the lump had been small, she had been too modest to show it to anyone. Now, since it had become worse, she consulted Democedes.

In the *Apocrypha*, in the Second Book of Maccabees, there is a dramatic account of what is presumed to be a carcinoma of the rectum, 'the Lord Almighty, the God of Israel, smote Antiochus with an incurable and invisible plague; a pain of the bowels that was remediless came upon him and sore torments of the inner parts. And while he lived in sorrow and pain, his flesh fell away and the filthiness of his smell was noisome to all his army' (Rendle Short 1953).

In more recent times, 1821, we can read an interesting account of the last illness of Napoleon. 'Napoleon's terminal illness lasted for six months. The history is quite clear: during his last days he suffered from tarry stools and coffee grounds vomit, both of which appearances are caused by digested or semi-digested blood. The post-mortem reports vary as to the condition of Napoleon's liver, but all mention a large scirrhous growth of the stomach. This with the above history make the diagnosis and cause of death quite certain. Napoleon died from a cancer of the stomach, which had pierced the wall, leaving an aperture sufficiently large to admit a finger. The cancer had eroded a blood vessel; death was due to exhaustion from haemorrhage and peritonitis resulting from perforation of the stomach by the malignant growth. His end was a merciful one, for he might have lingered on to die from sheer starvation (Cartwright, 1972).'

From the history of the disease we pass to the history of treatment. Probably no other disease has given rise to such bizarre treatments and, even today, this continues. As already indicated, the earliest forms of treatment were primitive in the extreme, and many involved the cult of witchcraft and superstition. Old-fashioned herbal books describe many concoctions for cure and relief of 'cankers'. Galen described the doctrine of the four humours and taught 'that people in whom black bile predominated were liable to develop tumours, as the bile tended to solidify in certain elective sites such as the lips, breast and tongue. Cancer was thus an internal disease which had to be treated by purgatives'.

In 1757 a French surgeon, Le Dean, postulated a completely new theory that cancer was a local lesion which spread through the lymphatics and that it could recur. His theory was founded on his own findings in the post-mortem room. Percival Pott in 1775 described the cancers found in chimney sweeps and in 1806 the *Edinburgh Medical and Surgical Journal* published the original questionnaire to define current thoughts on cancer.

Causation of cancer

There is no single type of cancer, and therefore no single cause. Many theories have been put forward and substantiated by research, and although it is not possible to go into any of this in depth, it is nevertheless necessary to briefly review this immensely fascinating part of the whole mystery of cancer.

CARCINOGENS

Both physical factors such as X-rays and ultraviolet light rays, and chemical substances such as dyes, can convert normal cells into cancer cells. In 1775 Percival Pott noted that there was a considerable amount of scrotal cancer amongst chimney sweeps and attributed this to contact with soot. It was left to Kennaway in the 1920s to prove this. Physiotherapists will know that ankylosing spondylitis is sometimes treated by radiotherapy and it is not uncommon later to find a basal cell carcinoma at the treatment site, in patients thus treated many years previously.

In rubber factories the use of dyes containing beta-naphthalene is now known to lead to cancer of the bladder in a significant proportion of cases, and its use is now forbidden. Wood dust from furniture-making leads to cancers of the sinuses, asbestos dust to lung cancer and cancers of the pleura, notably mesothelioma, and it is now required by law that masks or other protective clothing must be supplied to workers. Cigarettes, because of their coal tar content, probably present the greatest carcinogenic risk because they are easily available to all (Roe, 1971).

VIRUSES

Much discussion has taken place about the role of viruses in the causation of cancer, and it is certainly possible to produce cancers in animals with them. The rapidly growing tumour of the jaw found in East Africa, known as Burkitt's lymphoma, has been postulated by the discoverer, Denis Burkitt, to be due to a virus.

It may be that the virus acts as a trigger to set off some chain reaction which leads to the development of cancer. It may be that it is part of the process of the immunological response. Certainly a number of patients suffering from advanced cancer develop herpes zoster (shingles), which is caused by a virus. It is believed that herpes zoster is more likely to occur when the natural immunity of the body breaks down, and becomes apparent along the nerve roots of affected areas.

ENVIRONMENTAL AND DIETARY FACTORS

Studies among migrants from Japan to the United States have shown that environmental factors appear to influence the incidence of cancer. In particular the study of Haenszel and Kurihara (1968) shows that the mortality from stomach cancer of Japanese men and women living in Japan is much higher than that in white

A GENERAL BACKGROUND TO CANCER

citizens of the United States. When Japanese go to live in the United States, however, their risk of developing stomach cancer, and the risk of their children developing it, falls dramatically towards the level of the white citizen in the United States.

Burkitt (1972) has postulated that natives of African countries (who have a low incidence of bowel cancer) are more likely to develop bowel cancer when they become westernised because they stop eating foods containing cereal fibre. Here we might remember the words of Hippocrates, who wrote, 'To the human body it makes a great difference whether the bread is made of fine flour or corn, whether of wheat with the bran, or wheat without the bran'.

In Asian countries the habit of chewing betel nut or tobacco wrapped in lime contributes to the high incidence of mouth cancers.

Eskimos and Laplanders are known to have a high incidence of stomach cancer, and this has been attributed to eating fish cooked over smoke fires.

PREDISPOSING FACTORS

It is known that certain medical conditions may predispose a patient to develop cancer, and these people should be regularly checked.

(1) Familial adenosis (a condition of the colon characterized by multiple polyps) and ulcerative colitis both predispose towards cancer of the colon and rectum.

(2) Hiatal hernias, unless treated, produce oesophagitis which in turn can lead to a cancerous condition.

(3) Pitch warts occur in workmen exposed to tar and pitch, and fishermen who handle tarred ropes can develop pitch warts on their hands and arms. They should be excised because they may turn into malignant conditions in later years.

(4) Systemic lupus erythematosus and dermatomyositis may be the first signs of a silent carcinoma.

Prevention and control

From the preceding paragraphs it will be seen that many cancers may be caused through contact with certain noxious stimuli and the avoidance of such contact should diminish the risk of developing the disease.

It is interesting to note that substances such as the aromatic amines, e.g. beta-naphthylamine, are now by Act of Parliament forbidden to be used in those industries that formerly used them. Protective clothing, as already mentioned, must be supplied to workers in the asbestos and furniture and allied wood-turning industries, and this includes the provision of respirators where necessary.

The *Radiation Protection Act* lays down stringent rules regarding the safety of all personnel engaged in work where radiation is likely. Radiologists and radiographers wear lead aprons when screening patients in diagnostic units, and in radiotherapy units all treatment rooms are lead-lined.

EARLY SCREENING AND EDUCATION

Where it is known that there is a risk, regular screening of personnel should be carried out. This should take place in working hours and form part of the employer's responsibility towards his workers. Patients with a family history of cancer should undergo regular checks.

A great deal of education in a general way is taking place. The keynote to success lies in the ability to stress the hopeful nature of the treatment of cancer, provided that early diagnosis is made. Breast and cervical examinations are now freely available throughout the country and need take only a very short time. Education is something in which the physiotherapist can play a very active part, and this will be dealt with in Chapter Twelve. To sum up, education, and consequently early screening, plus the avoidance of known cancer-inducing substances, could go a long way towards reducing the mortality lists.

Pathology

To understand the cancerous diseases sufficiently to be able to be more effective in the approach to patients, it is helpful if the physiotherapist appreciates the fundamental histological and pathological forms of tumours. This basic understanding will lead to a more perceptive insight into what must be described as a fascinating group of diseases.

The normal cell can be viewed quite simply as consisting of a nucleus surrounded by cytoplasm. Both the nucleus and the cytoplasm are delicately balanced with a make-up of chemical compounds. It is when this balance is upset that the reproduction of the cell does not follow its normal pattern. When the cell starts becoming unbalanced, a tumour will grow. What triggers off this imbalance is not known. It would appear that there is no single cause; research indicates that it may be due to chemical carcinogens, dietary or other factors in the environment, viruses or a combination of these. One essential feature of the cancer cell is that it is capable of division, sometimes rapidly and sometimes more slowly, but it does not reach maturity and is said to be anaplastic.

TUMOURS

A tumour is a lump which may develop in any part of the body. It is composed of newly developed cells which are derived from the normal cells of the body, and these cells may possess microscopical resemblance to normal cells. The rate at which the cells divide will decide how rapidly the tumour grows. Tumours are either benign or malignant, and are differentiated by their behaviour.

BEHAVIOUR OF MALIGNANT TUMOURS

(1) They grow rapidly, although slow growth does not necessarily indicate a benign tumour (e.g. rodent ulcer, where growth is very slow).

(2) They invade neighbouring tissues.

(3) They invade blood and lymph vessels and thus cancer cells can spread to other structures causing metastases.

(4) They can recur locally after removal. This must be remembered when surgical removal is carried out, and the excision must be wide enough so that the edges are well clear of tumour.

The site of the tumour may determine how early symptoms are presented, e.g. a cancer may grow to an enormous size in the stomach, before symptoms show, because it is a hollow organ. On the other hand a cancer of the lung which impinges on a main bronchus and produces acute breathlessness should be promptly diagnosed and can be quite small.

METASTASES

A metastasis is a secondary tumour which develops at a distance from the primary tumour but has characteristics that are microscopically identical. Metastases can appear early or late in the natural history of the tumour, and it is well-known that certain cancers will metastasise to well-recognized areas: for example, a breast cancer to bone and lymph nodes, bronchial cancer to the other lung or the brain, bone sarcoma to lungs, alimentary tract cancer to the liver. Sometimes a metastasis may be the first symptom which brings a patient to hospital, for example a pathological fracture of femur may lead to a minute breast cancer being found. Nowadays metastases can be discovered by means of scinti-scanning even before they are evident on an X-ray.

DIFFERENTIATION OF TUMOURS

Tumours may be described histologically as differentiated and non-differentiated. A tumour is differentiated when the cells are arranged in such a pattern that one can differentiate the organ of origin. These tumours are usually regarded as relatively slow-growing. When a tumour is non-differentiated or anaplastic (both words have the same meaning), the cells are arranged in a disorganized manner with variation in size and shape and more frequent mitoses. Such tumours are said to be rapidly growing and tend to spread more rapidly and may therefore be regarded as more malignant. It is sometimes impossible to determine the organ of origin because the histological pattern is devoid of any order or arrangement.

Classification and staging of tumours

Attempts are made to classify tumours so that a prognostic estimation for a particular patient is possible, as well as providing a means of comparing different methods of treatment for different tumour stages. Obviously this classification must be universal and such a classification is that known as the TNM staging.

This is a method devised by the International Union against Cancer and the principles are straightforward and simple.

T stands for Tumour.
N stands for the regional lymph Nodes.
M stands for the distant Metastases.

By the addition of numbers to the three letters, e.g. T_1, T_2, T_3, N_1, M_2, different sizes of tumour and different degrees of the spread of disease are indicated, and from the build-up of the TNM code, the staging of the disease may be assessed. Though the tumour itself may be T_1, if there are any metastases the stage will always be 4.

This method of classification is based solely on clinical examination and has no bearing on subsequent histological examination. However simple and accurate such a method may be, there are still many indefinable factors which may influence the prognosis. These factors include the histological differentiation, the tumour-host or immunotherapeutic relationship, the time lapse between discovery of symptoms and seeking advice, and, of course, there is always the response to treatment by the tumour.

All of us can site cases of a so-called early cancer or stage 1 cancer that has progressed rapidly, and the patient has died within a short time, whilst stage 4 disease or advanced cancers may respond to treatment in dramatic ways.

Chapter Two: **A general outline of diagnostic methods**

Clinical diagnosis

An accurate diagnosis is essential for the treatment of a patient with a suspected malignant tumour. The first thing that is done when a patient reaches the consultant on referral from the family doctor, will be the taking of a *full* and searching history, including family background, social habits and occupation, proceeding to the signs and symptoms which prompted the patient to seek advice. It is worth while spending considerable time at this initial consultation for by it a good rapport may be established from the beginning between doctor and patient.

The taking of a history will be followed by a clinical examination which, again, will be thorough and not restricted to the local area. This clinical examination may include palpation of the tumour, particularly if it is accessible, and endoscopic examinations, particularly sigmoidoscopy and proctoscopy for rectal and colonic lesions, and indirect laryngoscopy for throat lesions.

Clinical examinations may also include blood tests, bone marrow examination, X-ray examination, isotope scanning. Physiotherapists should form the habit of reading the case-history of all patients referred to them for treatment, for they may often pick up some item of information which could influence their approach to the patient.

Special diagnostic facilities. A number of specialized diagnostic facilities are available which enable an earlier and more accurate diagnosis to be made. Physiotherapists may well be asked by patients what to expect when they undergo these examinations, and it cannot be emphasized too much that the physical treatment of all patients is far more interesting and rewarding if the principles of other facets of their treatment are understood.

MAMMOGRAPHY

This is a soft tissue X-ray of the breasts in which industrial film is used; two views of each breast are taken, a lateral and a craniocaudal. Carcinomas as small as 0·5 cm can be demonstrated. Tiny calcified flecks seen on a mammogram are strongly indicative of a carcinoma. Mammography does use X-rays and for this reason there must be a certain hazard if repetitive screening of a patient is carried out, particularly on women under 50 (Gillbe, 1973).

XEROGRAPHY

By definition, xerography is the science of duplicating graphic material and xeroradiography is the science of recording radiographic images photo-electrically. An electrostatically charged selenium-coated plate is used instead of the conventional X-ray film. The plate is used in precisely the same way as for a mammogram. The finished print is a positive in blue and white with well-defined edges and clear-cut detail. Lesions of about 2 mm can be detected. As these would certainly be impalpable, there is cautious optimism that this diagnostic facility could be of considerable use for the detection of early breast cancer. Considerable research on these comparable diagnostic methods has been carried out in the United States (Wolfe, Dooley & Hawkins, 1971). Xerography can also be used for bone and soft tissue examination. (See Plates 1 and 2 for xeroradiograph of a normal breast and one of a breast containing a cancer.)

THERMOGRAPHY

This is the production of a regional temperature map, particularly of the breast. By means of an infra-red camera, it is possible to record as a photograph the temperature of the area. To carry out this examination it is necessary for the patient to be first cooled; for breast examination the patient strips to the waist and sits with her arms resting comfortably at shoulder height so that there can be a free flow of air over all areas. It takes up to 20 minutes for the area which has been in contact with clothes to cool sufficiently so that false positives are reduced to a minimum (Holt, 1973). A cancerous area will be at a higher temperature than its surrounds and will show as a black area on the picture. Thermography is not as accurate as mammography or xerography but it has the great advantage of being quite safe.

LYMPHOGRAPHY AND ANGIOGRAPHY

These are radiological procedures in which various radio-opaque media are injected to enable detailed examination of specific vessels and organs.

Lymphography entails the injection of opaque medium into a lymph vessel and is a minor surgical procedure carried out by a radiologist under local anaesthesia. It may be carried out on a lymphoedematous arm to ascertain whether the lymphatic system is still patent or whether it has become disorganized. For arms, the incision is usually on the dorsum of the hand and if there is gross oedema involving the hand, the examination will almost certainly not be possible. For a pelvic and lower limb examination, the incision will be on the dorsum of the foot. In both cases, the examination requires two visits on consecutive days, which allows time for the medium to be taken up by the nodes; serial follow-up X-rays may be taken over many months from the time of the initial injection and thus it enables a check to be kept on the efficacy of any treatment which may be carried out. Patients should be reassured that their urine will be a brilliant green following the examination and it is probably useful for the physiotherapist to know this, so that she is in a position to reassure if necessary. Any physiotherapy treatment which may have been in progress for a lymphoedematous arm or leg should be suspended until the incision has healed.

DIAGNOSTIC METHODS

If nodes are affected by disease, they will not take up the dye in the same way as normal nodes and the position of nodes with filling defects will enable doctors to assess the extent of disease. (See Plates 3 and 4 for a normal lymphogram and the typical filling defects of nodes affected by a follicular lymphoma.)

Angiography. This entails the injection of contrast media into various blood vessels to aid diagnosis. The most common is probably an intravenous pyelogram, when an iodine medium is injected in the cubital fossa to outline the kidneys and urinary system. Cerebral angiography may be used in the diagnosis of cerebral tumours; a phlebogram may be carried out on a lymphoedematous arm to show whether the axillary vein is patent.

X-ray diagnostic techniques are becoming increasingly important in the diagnosis of malignant tumours, and physiotherapists working in this field of medicine would find it very useful to spend a short time in their respective X-ray departments seeing some of these examinations.

ISOTOPE SCANNING

Isotope scanning has developed very rapidly in the last five years and it is now possible to scan virtually the whole person for evidence of disseminated disease. The most usual sites for scanning are brain, bones, liver, thyroid and pancreas. The most commonly used isotope is technetium 99m (Tc^{99m}), because of its short half-life of 6 hours. 'Half-life' refers to the time taken for an isotope to decay to half its initial value.

The other commonly used isotope is iodine 131 (I^{131}).

The selected isotope is given in liquid form by an intravenous or oral route and the length of time before the examination that the isotope is administered will depend on the site to be scanned. The patient is placed in the optimum position and likewise the scinti scanner, which then moves back and forth over the area under examination (Simpson, 1974). Quite recently it has become normal practice in some centres to routinely body-scan all patients who have breast cancer in the possible chance of picking up early silent metastases.

CYTOLOGY

Cytology is the study of the formation and function of cells, and in the context of diagnosis, refers to the process of examining microscopically cells shed from the tumour surface and present in secretions. The obvious example of this procedure is the cervical smear, in which a wooden spatula is used to scrape the secretion present on the cervix or in the vagina, then carefully spread on a slide, and subsequently stained and examined under a microscope.

Other cytological examinations can be done on sputum, urine, pleural and peritoneal fluid and the washings from the stomach (Balmforth, 1948).

BIOPSY

Biopsy by definition means the microscopical examination of tissues taken from the body. In most cases a small piece of the suspect tumour is removed surgically and examined. In the field of breast surgery, a process has been devised whereby a biopsy may be taken and 'frozen' by a special technique, so that a rapid histological examination may be made and the answer conveyed to the surgeon within 15 minutes; if it is a positive result the surgeon is then able to proceed to major surgery at once and the patient does not have to endure a period of suspense. Where the initial examination is equivocal then it is necessary to proceed to a full sectioning of the biopsy, and this takes longer.

A biopsy may be taken by means of a drill, e.g. for breast and bone, a needle and aspiration, e.g. for lung or bone, a punch, e.g. for the cervix, or more usually with a scalpel. Biopsies may be taken either with or without anaesthetic, depending on the site. A biopsy is a very important part of the diagnostic facilities, for by the specimen's microscopical make-up the pathologist can determine whether the tumour is malignant, and also help to stage the tumour and determine its degree of malignancy.

Medical treatments for patients with a diagnosis of cancer

Once a diagnosis of cancer has been established, the plan of treatment has to be worked out. This requires teamwork, particularly if a combined approach to the disease is to be made. Within this team discussion, there may be occasion to consult the physiotherapist, the occupational therapist, and the social worker. From the beginning it is imperative that the whole person should be considered, and if radical surgery is to be performed, the need for reassurance about the future is essential. A woman will need to know that her husband and family will be helped where necessary; a man will need to be reassured about his ability to continue to be the breadwinner. The social worker can reassure and help from the social angle, the physiotherapist can reassure about walking if amputation is contemplated, about breathing if lung surgery is contemplated, or other relevant conditions.

The patient should be able to feel that everyone is concerned to help, and from the beginning he should be aware of all the services that can be mobilized to help him and his family at any time, and for as long as is necessary, if the need arises. It is noticeable that when patients and families are aware of all the help that is available, they seldom require it; the mere fact of knowing is often sufficient for presupposed problems to vanish.

The major lines of medical treatment which are available at the present time for the patient with cancer are chemotherapy, radiotherapy and surgery, which are discussed in Chapter Three.

Chapter Three: **An outline of medical and surgical treatments**

Surgery

Surgery still remains the main line of treatment when a diagnosis of cancer is made. Equally, most surgeons specializing in cancer treatments will work in combination with the radiotherapist and chemotherapist so that the best team approach can be made for each patient.

Great names in the historical roll of surgeons are still remembered today: Halsted and Patey for mastectomy; Wertheim for hysterectomy; Bilroth for gastrectomy; Miles for abdomino-perineal resection of rectum. Indeed Bilroth also performed the first recorded total laryngectomy in 1873 (Harrison, 1973).

Beatson of Glasgow, having had the chance to study lactation in sheep, noted in them the similarities of appearance of the growing mammary gland and breast cancer in women. This fact he remembered when he saw two women with advanced breast cancer. He reasoned that the removal of ovaries might remove the stimulus not only to the breast but possibly to the tumour as well. He removed the ovaries and noticed a dramatic improvement in one of the patients. Bilateral oophorectomy stands today as a standard procedure in advanced breast cancer as well as in prophylactic treatment by some surgeons in early cases.

The role of surgery, like other forms of treatment in the treatment of cancer, is either curative or palliative.

Curative surgery is carried out with the aim of removing the tumour in its entirety and can therefore be extremely extensive and, in some cases, very mutilating.

TYPES OF CANCERS AND SOME OF THE POSSIBLE OPERATIONS

Breast cancer
(1) *Halsted radical mastectomy.* This includes the whole breast, the pectoral muscles and a dissection of all axillary nodes. (A super-radical mastectomy may include a dissection of the internal mammary glands and the supraclavicular glands as well.)
(2) *Patey mastectomy.* Removal of the breast and axillary clearance without removal of pectoral muscles.
(3) *Simple mastectomy.* Removal of the bulk of breast tissue with a possible local axillary node dissection (this latter is not routine).

Stomach cancer
(1) Partial or total gastrectomy.
(2) Bypass procedures to relieve obstruction.

Oesophageal cancer
  Cervical region
Laryngo - pharyngo - oesophagectomy with tube replacement (skin or colon).

  Middle and lower third
(1) Oesophagectomy with stomach replacement.
(2) Intubation with various tubes, e.g. Owen's tube, Souttar's tube, Mousseau Barbin tube.

Lung Cancer
Thoracotomy proceeding to resection, either lobectomy or pneumonectomy.

Sarcoma of bone
Amputation depending on site but almost always very radical, e.g. forequarter, hindquarter, hemipelvectomy and disarticulation of shoulder and hip joints.

Kidney cancer
Nephrectomy.

Bladder cancer
Partial or total cystectomy with either

	transposition of ureters to rectum or the formation of an ileal conduit.
Rectal cancer	Abdominoperineal resection of rectum with formation of permanent colostomy, or anterior resection of rectum.
Colon cancer	Where possible, a right or left hemicolectomy or partial colectomy, but if too low, then anterior resection, or even an abdominoperineal resection.
Cancer of pancreas	(1) Whipple's operation. (2) Pancreatectomy. (3) Bypass procedures. (4) Insertion of gold grains to head of pancreas.
Cancers of head and neck	(1) Partial, hemi- or total glossectomy. (2) Partial or hemi-mandibulectomy with excision of floor of mouth, part of tongue plus repair of defect by grafting. (3) Partial or total maxillectomy plus exenteration of eye, depending on extent of disease.
Spinal cord tumours	Decompression laminectomy.

These are only some of the major operations and variations which may be encountered by physiotherapists. All are major, and all require the skill and help of all members of the caring team, including the physiotherapist. The full extent and exact procedure of these operations can be discovered by reference to any standard surgical text.

Palliative surgery is intended to relieve distressing and disabling sequelae of disease. It is essentially a humane approach to a difficult problem. A colostomy to relieve obstruction due to colonic cancer; a 'bypass' to relieve jaundice; a gastrostomy to enable a patient with complete oesophageal obstruction to be fed. These are obvious forms of palliative surgery, but there are other types which are worth mentioning since the physiotherapist is more than likely to find herself involved in their after-care and rehabilitation.

(1) Where metastatic disease affects the bones, pathological fractures can occur. These can be successfully pinned and treated, thus enabling the patient to become mobile instead of finding himself bedridden as in past times.

(2) Some tumours have been found to be hormone-dependent, and the patient who develops disseminated disease may be helped by surgical removal or ablation of one or other of the endocrine glands. This is particularly so in cases of disseminated breast cancer where bilateral adrenalectomy or hypophysectomy (removal of the pituitary gland) may have striking results.

(3) Advanced cancer may be accompanied by pain which can sometimes be almost intractable and not amenable to analgesics. Neurological surgeons can offer help in these cases, either by injection into the nerves carrying the pain impulses or by surgery involving division of the spinal tracts.

Radiotherapy

Radiotherapy is the treatment of malignant disease by the accurate use of penetrating radiations. In 1895 Röntgen discovered X-rays, in 1896 Becquerel discovered the radioactivity of uranium, and in 1898 Pierre and Marie Curie discovered radium. A whole range of radiotherapy treatments has developed from these early discoveries. It is not proposed to go into detail about the way in which these therapeutic radiations are produced or how they work, but a few short comments are necessary as background information.

Like radio waves, X-rays can be long, short or very short. The longer rays have only a superficial penetration and are used for treating skin tumours, e.g. rodent ulcers; as the wavelength decreases so the beam will penetrate to a greater depth, so that at the other extreme we have the linear accelerator and betatron which can treat deep-seated tumours, e.g. those of the bladder, bronchus and oesophagus, and yet not cause damage to the superficial tissues. The terms which will be used to describe these machines are:

superficial (60 to 140 kV), conventional (200 to 300 kV), and caesium, supervoltage, cobalt, linear accelerator up to 6 MeV and very high voltages up to 12 MeV. In addition newer equipment such as neutron therapy is now coming into use. These rays are all of the external variety and require accurate positioning of the tubes. With some tumours, particularly those of the head and neck, moulds or casts are made so that the patient's head is not allowed to wander and accuracy is made easier. Very careful planning for each patient is required and the exact dosage has to be worked out by the physicist and continually checked during treatment.

INTERNAL IRRADIATION

Internal irradiation may be achieved by the use of radioactive materials. Radium was the original of these substances to be used, being of a natural form, but since the end of the 1939-45 war, 'artificial' radioactive substances have been available from nuclear reactors. These include radioactive cobalt, caesium, gold, yttrium and others. As well as solid radioactive isotopes it is possible to get 'liquid' isotopes, i.e. isotopes in solution, e.g. iodine, gold and phosphorus. All these substances with the exception of radium have a definite life, i.e. the length of time they remain radioactive, and this should be appreciated by the physiotherapist. Radium is highly radioactive and virtually indestructible, i.e. its half-life is 1600 years! It is only left in situ for a comparatively short time and physiotherapy should *not* be given in this time unless by direct request from the consultant (Downie, 1971).

Internal irradiation may be effected by implanting the isotope in the form of needles, which are later removed, or by grains, which depending on the site will probably be permanently in situ. For carcinoma of the cervix it will be achieved by special intra-cavitary packs which are removed; for the pleura or peritoneum it will be by instillation direct into the cavity.

SIDE-EFFECTS

It must be emphasized at once that many patients undergoing

radiotherapy suffer no side-effects whatsoever. With rays of longer wavelength there is more likelihood of skin soreness, which is sometimes seen with post-mastectomy irradiation. Obviously fair-skinned people are more likely to suffer skin reactions. Occasionally the reaction can be severe enough to cause suspension of treatment; local applications which can be used include calamine lotion, calamine and tannic lotion, gentian violet, Betnovate cream, and many others depending on the consultant's views. In all cases the area must be kept dry and clean. For mastectomy patients a 'vest' cut out of Tubiton gauze will protect the chest from unnecessary rubbing. Nylon *must not* be worn next to a sore area.

Other side-effects which may occur will depend upon the area under treatment. They may include diarrhoea and vomiting, nausea, difficulty in swallowing, loss of taste, loss of hair (epilation), frequency of micturition and dysuria. The treatment of any of these will be essentially symptomatic, together with strong reassurance.

Types of case suitable for radiotherapy. As with chemotherapy, some tumours are primarily treated by radiotherapy, others in combination with other treatment and for others it is a form of palliative treatment.

PRIMARY TREATMENT

Conditions which are usually treated by radiotherapy as the major approach include Hodgkin's disease, which is a disease that affects the lymphatic system and is characterized by a particular cell which is discerned by histological examination, and other lymphomas, seminomas, basal cell and squamous cell carcinoma of the skin. Some tumours which cannot be removed surgically, e.g. certain brain tumours, will be treated primarily by radiotherapy. Likewise cancer of the larynx and cervix may also be treated initially by radiotherapy, depending upon the stage of the disease, and the desire not to inflict any more permanent damage than is necessary on the patient.

COMBINATION TREATMENT

Radiotherapy may be used as an adjunct to surgery, either pre- or postoperatively. This is particularly so with breast cancer, bladder cancer, bone sarcomas and others. Thus the radiotherapists in co-operation with a variety of surgeons (general, ear nose and throat, urological) will all work in harmony in order to provide the best possible chance for effective cure.

PALLIATIVE USE

Irradiation has a definite place in the treatment of metastases, e.g. bone metastases, inoperable soft tissue sarcomas, pathological fractures, and fungating ulcers. Relief of pain through irradiation of a bone metastasis can be quite dramatic and is fully justified as a means of treatment, even in a dying patient.

Chemotherapy

Treatment of tumours by cytotoxic drugs has made rapid advances over twenty-five years, and particularly in the last five years. It stems from the observation that nitrogen mustard, a lethal gas once used in warfare, produced a fall in the number of white blood cells, and subsequent clinical studies showed similar falls in the excess white blood cells of leukaemia (Bodley Scott, 1970).

From this beginning much research has gone into the screening of chemical compounds for effective use against human tumours. Today there are some thirty compounds which are to be found used in chemotherapy. Some are derived from plants, e.g. vincristine from the tropical periwinkle. Some are antibiotics, e.g. actinomycin D, whilst others are alkylating agents or antimetabolites. All these drugs will inhibit or destroy cancer cells, but their action is rarely specific to the cancer cell and therefore there will be damage to normal tissue.

Chemotherapy may be given as a single drug, but is more

usually given in combination groups, and the use of acronyms is a popular way of identifying many of these groups, e.g. MOPP (methotrexate, Oncovin (vincristine), procarbazine, prednisone) and FOME (5-fluorouracil, Oncovin, methotrexate, Endoxana (cyclophosphamide)).

Chemotherapy may be given orally, intravenously, or intramuscularly. It can also be given intra-arterially via an infusion and it has been given intrathecally where leukaemia cells have reached the central nervous system. Unfortunately these drugs do have side-effects, and it is useful to know about them, for they may well lead to an adjustment in treatments which physiotherapists may be giving at the same time.

SIDE-EFFECTS

Cyclophosphamide, used for chorion carcinoma and ovarian carcinoma, can lead to loss of hair (epilation) and it is essential that a wig is available *at once*. It is no good waiting until all the hair has fallen out and the patient very upset before arranging for a wig to be available. Patients need to be reassured that their hair will grow again, and the physiotherapist can weigh in with reassurance just as much as the nurse or doctor.

Methotrexate, used in chorion carcinoma, leukaemia, head and neck cancers, and bladder cancers, can lead to mouth ulceration and malabsorption.

Vincristine, used for leukaemia, reticuloses, and ovarian carcinoma, is neurotoxic and patients can develop paraesthesia and foot drop. Physiotherapists definitely need to look for this and indeed may be asked to treat patients because of the side-effects of this drug.

Other drugs used include 5-fluorouracil, vinblastine, actinomycin D, nitrogen mustard, melphalan, Bleomycin and many new ones which are appearing all the time. All these drugs cause a fall in the white blood count and consequently patients are more susceptible to infection. Gastric upsets are not uncommon and many of these patients feel very ill and miserable and need to be treated with compassion and understanding.

PRIMARY TREATMENT

Treatment with these drugs may indeed be curative in certain malignancies such as chorion epithelioma, a rare cancer which affects placental tissues (Bagshawe, 1972). It is now an impressive treatment for the leukaemias. Myelomatosis or plasmacytoma, a disease which affects the plasma cells and leads to bone deposits, is another type of cancer initially treated with drugs.

SUPPORTIVE TREATMENT

Chemotherapy is used to support other forms of treatment, and a common example is in the treatment of Wilms' tumour, a kidney tumour found in children. Here, radiotherapy is given with actinomycin D.

PALLIATIVE TREATMENT

When surgery is not feasible and where radiotherapy has been used to its maximum, chemotherapy may also have a place. Often this is in cases of advanced head and neck cancers, and the advantages and disadvantages need to be carefully weighed. Quality of extended life is infinitely more important than extended survival at all costs.

Immunotherapy

William Jenner is rightly considered the father of immunotherapy by his chance finding that infecting people with cowpox protected them against smallpox. Nowadays there is much interest in applying the principle of immunotherapy to the management of patients with cancer. Immunotherapy is simply the stimulating of the body's own defence mechanisms to react against a foreign substance, in this case the tumour.

Chapter Four: The philosophy of rehabilitation for cancer patients

The need for rehabilitation for patients with cancer is becoming increasingly accepted, particularly as the newer treatments and earlier diagnosis are enabling patients to live longer. For this reason the patient must be treated as a whole person with a body, mind and soul, and rehabilitation is not therefore a matter of physical treatment only. Neither must rehabilitation be thought of as a means of prolonging life. Many centuries ago, Plato said, 'For this is the great error of our day, that in treating of the human body, physicians separate the soul from the body', and in our own times the philosophy of rehabilitation has been described in the following words: 'Let the patient understand his disability, regain confidence and be inspired, always making sure that fears and anxieties are dispelled and that social problems are solved. Physical exercise alone is not rehabilitation, psychological and social treatment is just as important as active physical treatment' (Watson Jones, 1958).

Having defined rehabilitation as offering total care to the patient as a whole, the question of prognosis must also be considered. This is a loaded observation and any comment must be guarded. The question of prognosis is not part of a physiotherapist's work, but she must learn to assess her goals and her treatment in the light of an estimated prognosis. It is possible to think in terms of 'long' and 'short' prognoses and thus to adjust the approach accordingly. With experience and working with a team one becomes quite skilled in making an assessment, and even sometimes making it more accurately than the doctors. Obviously with a short prognosis the patient must be made as independent as possible without resource to sophisticated techniques. A long-term prognosis will allow for a more intensive and graded programme. 'Short' in this context means a matter of weeks, and 'long' a matter of years, but between these two groups there is an area where one does not know what the outcome may be, and these patients are those who must always be given the benefit of the doubt and thoroughly rehabilitated.

If rehabilitation is defined as total care, what then does this entail? Physiotherapy and rehabilitation are not synonymous, and the physiotherapist has a chance to develop other talents in understanding and meeting the needs of these patients. She must learn to work with all members of the team and be prepared to ask any one of them for help for the patient. Many of these patients will be very frightened and may well use the physiotherapist as a sympathetic listener. All sorts of problems may emerge and, whilst a patient's utterances must always be regarded as confidential, it may be necessary to ask his or her permission to seek the assistance of someone else more capable of helping. It must not be implied that one is not interested or that one has not the time. Sitting down and listening to a patient may well be the finest form of true rehabilitation and should never be regarded as a waste of time.

Usha Batt, discussing rehabilitation of cancer patients in India, has written, 'Till recent times it was customary for doctors to take into consideration only the medical or physical aspects of any disease including cancer. Today, however, they have realized that a human being is not just an assortment of organs and extremities. A cancer patient is not merely an individual with a diseased body; he is also a person with a throbbing heart, a thinking mind, a stirring soul and one who lives in a small world of his own, surrounded by his family and friends. He has a physical disease that can be treated by the doctor, but he also has attitudes and aptitudes; interests and instincts; hopes and dreams of the future—which are all affected by his malady.'

If then, through radical treatment, the disease is controlled or even cured, it follows that this will properly be adjudged as successful if the patient is still able to enjoy life, to return to work where applicable and to regain his place in society as a whole. It has truly been said that 'the society which fosters research to save human life cannot escape responsibility for the life thus extended. It is for science not only to add years to life, but more important, to add life to the years'.

Rehabilitation for the cancer patient, as indeed for other patients too, is a team effort and the physiotherapist needs to know what her co-equal supporting colleagues can offer for any patient receiving physiotherapy. Professional training can indeed be self-limiting. Exchanging roles, blurring professional lines of demarcation is not always easy. There is a very natural desire to apply acquired skills and techniques and to see results by one's own unaided efforts. This practice can lead to frustration and discouragement. The support of professional colleagues is vital in dealing with a complex situation (Hawker, 1974). A patient who undergoes laryngectomy will receive both chest physiotherapy and speech therapy; if the physiotherapist consults with her speech therapist colleague she can probably incorporate suitable breathing exercises into her treatment, thus giving the patient an added incentive to practise, in the knowledge that the exercises will help him to produce a new speech. This will also be helpful to the speech therapist. A patient who is to have a limb amputated will benefit greatly by meeting the limb fitter beforehand and learning what will be expected from him; likewise the physiotherapist will benefit from being included in this kind of discussion. But all this will only come about by joint discussion and meetings with various colleagues in order to discover how each can help the other to the best advantage of the patient.

Whilst the social worker is available to resolve special problems, she cannot do this if she does not know what is required. It may sometimes happen that a patient may express concern about financial, familial or business matters to the physiotherapist. It is for her to alert the social worker to the needs of that particular patient. When the time comes for the patient to leave hospital, there is continuing care at home to be considered. Often this requires considerable co-operation, and any member of the treatment team may be asked to act as co-ordinator between the hospital and community. Every member of the rehabilitation team must be willing to have a share in this, even if it does mean moving outside one's own allotted sphere of work. There must be no question of 'it's not my job', or 'I wasn't trained for this'. The needs of the patient are paramount and personal animosities must be set aside.

To be part of a rehabilitation team can be frustrating and difficult, but equally it can be richly rewarding. With cancer patients it can also have its moments of utter tragedy and sadness, and these are the times when it is essential that each member of the team supports the other, and one's philosophical approach is seen to advantage. Within the team will be found everyone who may have contact with the patient or his family; obviously they will not all be needed for every patient or all the time. A team will include, apart from the obvious medical, nursing and paramedical personnel, the chaplain, the ambulancemen, the hospital porter, the ward maid, the volunteer, the district nurse, the home help and many others. But at the heart of every team is the patient and he is as much part of the team as anyone else. In many cases, as physiotherapists well know, it is the patient who dictates the progress and the goals set. If the right result is achieved, then that is satisfactory, but if it looks as though the plan is going astray then a discussion together will usually lead to a more realistic approach. The patient should at all times be kept in the picture and the best way to do this is to discuss with him how to achieve objects. It is unwise to tell some patients they will not be able to do this, that or the other. It is far better to let them try and find out for themselves that they cannot, and then they are much more likely to accept your suggestion on another occasion.

Many frustrations for both a patient and his family stem from being kept in the dark. Rehabilitation will only be successful if one has the co-operation of the patient and his family and it therefore follows that mutual discussion must be advantageous.

One hopes always that rehabilitation will end in return to work or a good life at home, but sometimes it ends in death and this should be realized by the people treating the patient. If a patient clearly deteriorates, it is quite wrong to withdraw all active care. Obviously it has to be modified and adapted, but to help a patient accept his death and to support relatives through this period, is as much rehabilitation as restoring him to a full life in this world. Physiotherapists need to be aware of this and be prepared to play their part in care for the dying patient.

When the British Council for the Rehabilitation of the Disabled was founded in 1944, the founders defined rehabilitation as 'the whole range of services from the time of onset of the individual's disability to the point at which he is restored to normal activity or the nearest possible approach to it'. To this should be added 'or until he dies'. Rehabilitation in essence is total patient care by many people including the physiotherapist and it should continue, particularly for cancer patients, from the moment of diagnosis to the ultimate end. Indeed for many cancer patients and in particular those who have disseminated disease or those who are suffering from varying paralyses, active rehabilitation will continue for many years, through both good and difficult patches.

Clearly the physiotherapist must come to terms with the implication of a diagnosis of cancer. The result may indeed be death, but this must not be allowed to diminish the physiotherapist's enthusiasm for treating the patient. Because of the nature of cancerous diseases quite unexpected results do occur, and the patient must therefore be approached with a positive attitude.

Cancer is an emotive word, for to many it spells grief, despair, bewilderment, fury, frustration and indeed the whole range of human emotions. It is therefore imperative that all who have close contact with cancer patients should fashion out their own general philosophy: one must be sympathetic without being sentimental, one must be practical without being hardhearted, one must be able to impart hope when all seems black, one must be willing to listen and one must know when to keep silent and when to seek help.

Fashioning such a philosophy is not an easy matter: it is learnt with experience in treating such patients, in learning from the example of others who are practised in the art of caring, and patient understanding. Not least does it come from the courageous way in which so many patients with a cancerous disease accept the diagnosis, and with it the challenge to live their lives as fully as possible.

Only with such a philosophy is it possible to begin to understand the fears expressed by so many patients, and by so doing to help them face these fears and to see them in true perspective. This underlines the importance of listening. Quite often it is of more value to listen and talk to patients, seeking to understand their fears, troubles, hopes and expectations, than it is to blindly accept a diagnosis and treat that alone, without giving due thought to what the particular patient wishes to do in the future.

CASE-HISTORY

The following case-history admirably illustrates this. Mr. V. was a man of 40 with an osteochondroma of the upper end of the right femur. He received pre-operative irradiation and then a disarticulation of the hip was carried out. Pre-operatively he had been trained in the use of elbow crutches and taught to walk and manage stairs. Postoperatively he received leg exercises to maintain the muscle strength of the left leg and as soon as the drains were removed (fifth day) he was mobilized on crutches. He was very quickly ambulant and completely independent; within three weeks he was referred for the initial fitting of a Canadian-type tilting-table prosthesis. The fittings and preliminary walking training were carried out at a limb fitting centre. During this time the patient expressed to the original physiotherapist that as he was a devout Roman Catholic he wished more than anything else to be able to kneel at the altar rails and to genuflect without the aid of sticks. Thus, it was possible to arrange for the last and most important part of his rehabilitation to be carried out in the hospital chapel so as to ensure that his wish was fulfilled (see Plate 5). A happy and contented patient left the hospital after major treatment, secure in the knowledge that he was fully rehabilitated.

Apart from demonstrating the rewards which come with listening, this case-history also illustrates the importance of the physiotherapist establishing a good rapport with the patient. Whilst this is necessary for all good treatment, it is vitally important with the patient suffering from cancer because the treatment programme may be very long and may even extend periodically over many years. The patient will look for, and expect, help, confidence and integrity, and there must be mutual trust and respect. Much of this will be expressed in the way the physiotherapist handles the patient. The firm confident grip and support for a painful joint or limb may give greater reassurance to a patient than pious platitudes uttered at the bedside. It is often important to give a short and sensible explanation as to why the treatment is essential, for patients do not like being treated as children or idiots. Particularly is this true of those who have suffered brain tumours and whose intellect is unimpaired, but whose reactions are slowed.

As one considers the approach to these patients it should be remembered that whilst the physiotherapist may be treating a specific part, it may in fact be only a local manifestation of a generalized condition. This is well demonstrated in the patient with a pathological fracture of the femur due to a metastasis from a primary breast cancer. Such patients may be receiving systemic treatment for their cancer and in consequence be in a poor general state of health. This is not a reason for postponing physiotherapy but it will certainly have a bearing on it. A table of exercises to tone up the general musculature together with specific leg exercises should be initiated as soon as the fracture has been stabilized (usually by intra-medullary pinning). As the general state of the patient improves, mobilization becomes possible. This type of patient presents a challenge which must be accepted, for they are very rewarding to treat.

The fact that a physiotherapist is treating such a patient will in itself be a boost to morale. Long-term medical treatment is not always pleasant, and with a fractured leg it becomes worse. The author is well aware of the despair and depression which surrounds such patients, and equally how cheered they can be by an explanation that pinning will soon enable them to be activated again. Indeed, many of these patients will have several years of good life ahead, and to a woman with a husband and a growing family every year is precious. It is therefore vital that all concerned in her treatment should give as much encouragement and support as possible.

It is also important that the physiotherapist meets the family,

PHILOSOPHY OF REHABILITATION

for often she is the best person to help them to rearrange the home to the best advantage, yet without making it totally unacceptable to the patient. The relatives can be shown how to offer unobtrusive help without appearing over-protective. They are thus enabled to play their part, and this goes a long way to preventing feelings of guilt which are often apparent as a patient's condition deteriorates.

The team approach

For many years a team approach, including the physiotherapist, has been utilized in the treatment of orthopaedic patients, and extended to the provision of peripheral clinics like that pioneered by Robert Jones and Agnes Hunt at Oswestry. In recent years the team approach to the patient suffering from a cancerous disease has been advocated, so that they are enabled to have the best co-ordinated treatment possible. This team may consist of a surgeon, general physician, radiotherapist and chemotherapist together with the necessary ancillary services. The ancillary services should include a nursing sister, physiotherapist, medical social worker, occupational therapist, speech therapist, prosthetic fitter, therapy radiographer, and chaplain. Not all will be required for each patient, but when they are required they should be included in the case discussion so that each of them knows exactly what is being planned for the patient, and more particularly what has been said to the patient. Who leads the team is a matter of opinion, but it is reasonable to expect that the consultant to whom the patient was first referred should act as leader. What is important, though, is that the team *and* the patient should know who is the leader.

Ideally, the physiotherapist should be present at the initial consultation if she is going to be involved to a great degree, for example if the patient is going to undergo extensive head and neck surgery, amputation, mastectomy, or radiotherapy following laminectomy for paraplegia. She then knows the patient before admission, and possibly meets the family as well; she has established her place and if it is apparent to the patient that there is a good rapport between consultant and physiotherapist, he will approach his admission with a more confident feeling. The relationship between patient and physiotherapist may become very close but must not be allowed to become emotional. A professional bearing must be maintained at all times. Once emotion and passion become apparent the physiotherapist will be in no position to give positive help to the patient and in such cases the author feels that the physiotherapist should if possible withdraw, and allow a colleague to take over. Emotion clouds the judgement and does not allow for an objective assessment; sentiment may allow one to let a patient accept a situation when sensibility would make one encourage the patient once again to fight and win another reprieve. This does not mean harrassing a patient who is dying or has really turned his face to the wall, but it does mean being extremely firm with a recalcitrant patient. Here again, if there is good rapport the patient will respect the firmness of the physiotherapist and the relationship will be strengthened.

The most difficult question of all, perhaps, is whether a patient should be told that he has a cancerous disease. This does not directly involve the physiotherapist, for the ultimate answer rests with the consultant, but no-one concerned with the treatment of cancer patients can escape discussion of this question. In theory this point should present no greater problem in cancer patients than in those with cardiac conditions, but in practice the fact that cancer as a diagnosis invariably equates with death in the minds of the general public, leads to much heart-searching. Some consultants would like the word 'cancer' abandoned and replaced by other terms, e.g. oncological diseases, tumours, etc., but whatever is done in the future, the truth remains today that cancer, despite many advances, is still the second commonest cause of death and people are frightened by the word.

With all this in mind, whatever is told to the patient *must* be accompanied by hope and reassurance at all times. Lies must not be told; equally it is not always necessary to tell the whole truth. It is possible to tell a patient that he has a tumour which may become very serious if it is not removed; it is possible to tell him that he has an ulcer which is best treated with rays. Experience and personal intuition is the only guide on how much is told. It is, however, important that the physiotherapist knows what the patient has been told, so that she is able to answer any further questions which may be put to her.

Some consultants will always tell the patient the complete truth of the immediate situation, coupling it with hope, confidence and reassurance. This makes for easier relations at the beginning, but as the disease makes relentless progress it has to be handled with great skill. Those patients who have a deep faith and who can and do accept the situation will teach and inspire those who treat them. There is no doubt that in all patients it is possible to sow the seed of truth of the future and then allow them to accept it, each according to his ability. But, if a lie is told, and the patient finds out, he will no longer trust anyone in the team and future treatment will be exceedingly difficult. Physiotherapists who are directly asked awkward questions should be able to look a patient squarely in the eyes and humbly answer 'I don't know'.

Chapter Five: **The role of physiotherapy in the treatment of patients receiving chemotherapy**

Chemotherapy, in this context, is the treatment of a patient suffering from a cancerous disease with carcinostatic drugs, which may be given systemically or locally.

Systemic chemotherapy

The drugs that are used not only destroy the tumour cells but they also destroy blood cells and damage the bone marrow and consequently cause a fall in the number of red or white corpuscles in the circulation. As a result, patients on systemic chemotherapy are at greater risk of infection and are liable to be in a rather debilitated state.

Many patients, particularly those with leukaemia or choriocarcinoma, are nursed in sterile units, and if physiotherapy is required for them (and this is by no means a routine requirement), the physiotherapist will have to acquaint herself with the precautions necessary before approaching the patient. Mostly this will entail some form of protective clothing, for the protection of the patient, *not* the physiotherapist. Sometimes this may be only mask, gown and overshoes, but in certain sterile units it will mean stripping, bathing and putting on completely sterile clothing before entering the patient's room. This is a time-consuming operation and it may be more practicable to teach the nursing staff (who have to be with the patient frequently) how to carry out the specific techniques.

General principles of treatment for patients receiving chemotherapy

(1) To maintain lung capacity and to clear secretions, thus helping to prevent unnecessary chest infections.
(2) To maintain joint mobility and to aid circulation, thus helping to prevent deformity and thrombosis.
(3) To maintain adequate muscle power.
(4) Where possible to maintain good posture.

CHEST PHYSIOTHERAPY

Many of these patients are acutely ill, and in consequence are not able to stand long or tiring treatments. Vibrations, change of position and good general deep breathing exercises would be the treatment of choice. When the nursing staff are treating the pressure areas is usually a good time to combine the physiotherapy treatment. Thus the patient is not subjected to two separate treatments, and the nursing staff can see what is being done by the physiotherapist and will know how to carry it out each time they treat the pressure areas. If a patient is too ill to stand manual vibrations, and yet has secretions, it may be sufficient to shake the mattress, thus applying indirect vibrations, to roll the patient gently, or to apply manual manipulation above the sternal notch.

As the patient's general condition improves, so physiotherapy may be increased to include gentle postural drainage of any specifically affected lobes and more specific breathing exercises with manual pressure to aid expansion.

In no circumstances must the patient be over-tired.

JOINT MOBILITY AND AID TO CIRCULATION

In weak and debilitated patients, joints must be carefully handled (Downie, 1973). Daily passive movements may be necessary to maintain joint range if the patient is too ill to move them himself. Nurses should be shown how to handle limbs so that as they turn the patient they do not drag the legs and put strain on weak joints. Gentle massage with oil will also help to relieve the discomfort of limbs which cannot easily be moved actively, and the oil will also help to keep the skin in a more supple state. Particular attention should be paid to maintaining good mobility of the toe and foot joints and the finger and wrist joints. If passive movements are adequately performed the joint range will be maintained, thus avoiding the use of splints which on weak and very ill patients can increase their discomfort. The passive movements and oil massage will help the circulation and help to prevent venous stasis and consequent thrombosis.

MAINTENANCE OF MUSCLE POWER

The amount of exercise which one can give patients on systemic chemotherapy will depend entirely on their condition. If they are able to move by themselves, then simple bed exercises such as static quadriceps contractions, foot dorsi- and plantar flexion, foot circling, toe flexion and extension, knee flexion and extension, should be encouraged. The upper limbs are best exercised by the patient performing, where possible, the normal activities of eating, drinking and washing. Some assistance will probably be required, but encouragement should be given to him to try. As soon as possible, one full range of active shoulder extension, internal and external rotation should be insisted upon each day. As for a Colles fracture, this is best done by asking the patient to raise his hand straight above his head, then scratch the back of his neck and finally to put his hand behind his back. Both arms may be exercised together or they may be worked singly, again depending upon the state of the patient.

MAINTENANCE OF GOOD POSTURE

This is not very easy to carry out on a weak and ill patient, but it can be helped by correct positioning of pillows so that the patient's back is fully supported with the head in a comfortable mid-position and not allowed to be pushed forward into flexion or to fall back into extension. A foot-board across the bottom of the cradle will help to maintain ankle dorsiflexion and will also help the patient to retain positional sense. It is sometimes forbidden to put pillows under knees because it leads to venous thrombosis as well as joint contractures. This is indeed so if the pillow is large and hard; however, a small towel lightly rolled and placed under the knees will give relief from aching. Provided it is replaced from time to time and a full range of joint mobility maintained, it will do no harm. As the patient improves, so postural correction can be carried out sitting over the side of the bed preparatory to standing (*Physiotherapy Helps Nursing*, 1962).

Rehabilitation for chemotherapy patients after the acute phase is over

As the general condition of a patient improves, active exercises may be increased. Here, it should be repeated, the physiotherapist is not often invited to help these patients, but when she is, she will be told at what stage the patient may leave his sterile surroundings. As soon as this can occur, the patient should be brought to the physiotherapy department and if possible work with others, so that he can begin to feel once more part of a normal environment.

Graded exercises will be given, working up to discharge from hospital for a spell at either a specific rehabilitation centre or a convalescent home and finally back to work—that is the final goal.

Many patients of this type will only have a short remission before returning for further intensive treatment, equally, others will have long periods of comparatively good health during which time they will hold down good jobs, or in the case of married women, continue to look after their husbands and families. Whatever the result, those who have received help and rehabilitation all through their illness will be better able to cope. From experience in a rehabilitation unit for patients with cancer who have been referred from many hospitals, it has been made abundantly plain that if only they had received some form of physiotherapy, most of the patients would indeed have been able to cope from an earlier point; the commonest remark to be heard is always: 'Why could I not have had this treatment when I was in hospital?'

CASE-HISTORY

The following case-history describes the rehabilitation for a patient prior to her discharge home.

Miss C. was a lady in her late forties, with chronic lymphatic leukaemia, treated with systemic chemotherapy. She was a secretary in the Foreign and Commonwealth Office. Previously she had been in good health, until 1969 when she had begun to feel less well and complained of frequent chest infections and mouth ulcers. Finally she had woken one morning to find that she could not see. She was referred to an eye hospital where acute anaemia was diagnosed and blood transfused. She continued to develop chest infections, and finally, on being fully investigated, was found to be suffering from chronic lymphatic leukaemia.

She received transfusions and was started on a chemotherapeutic regime of chlorambucil and prednisone. While in hospital she received no physiotherapy and prior to discharge it was felt she required some form of rehabilitative convalescence.

On admission she was assessed by both the consultant and the physiotherapist.

22 March 1971. On examination, general condition quite good, though looked strained. Muscle power good. Co-ordination poor and complained of unsteadiness and dizziness.

Treatment plan. (1) *General.* General limbering up classwork. Indoor games sessions. Aids to daily living, particularly household activities.

(2) *Specific.* (a) Intensive Frenkel's exercises to help co-ordination. (b) Specific strengthening exercises for legs and back. (c) General breathing exercises.

(3) *Social.* Encouragement to go down to town and do any shopping for other patients.

Observation. Miss C. told the physiotherapist that she had elderly parents and her main worry was for them; it was obvious then that all rehabilitation must be geared towards ability to run the house as well as helping her regain confidence to return to work.

5 April 1971. Great improvement noted. Co-ordination better and virtually no dizziness. Feels much better and wishes to try a weekend at home. (Miss C. had worked extremely hard with her exercises and could be found with squares marked out on the floor so that she could do her Frenkel's exercises whenever she had a spare moment!)

19 April 1971. For discharge home. Able to walk to town comfortably and back (one mile). No dizziness. Co-ordination now normal and had no complaints.

To be followed up at referring hosptial and to return to work as soon as possible.

June 1971. Returned to work on short hours. Continued physical improvement and increase of weight. Able to look after home and parents as well.

February 1972. Very fit and full-time working, 9.30 to 6.30, plus looking after parents. Continues with regular follow-up appointments and maintenance chemotherapy treatment.

May 1973. Continues very well.

This case-history admirably illustrates how a debilitated patient following chemotherapy can be rehabilitated with simple disciplined physiotherapy and help, reassurance and enthusiastic encouragement.

Simple classwork with other patients serves a dual purpose of providing exercise as well as a competitive spirit, and often it is the other patients who provide the impetus to recovery.

Chemotherapy by local infusion or perfusion

Sometimes a local tumour mass may be treated by an infusion of the specific drug direct into the artery which supplies the tumour area. Head and neck tumours are particularly amenable to this form of chemotherapy. A cannula is introduced into the artery, attached to a pump which in turn is attached to the drip containing the drug. Although only a local area is being treated, the blood count may drop dramatically and breathing exercises are usually given to prevent the onset of a chest infection. A quite violent local reaction can occur and patients may feel very ill for a short time. If the physiotherapist is involved with the patient she can offer encouragement to move gently and also reassure him that the reaction will be short-lived.

In the case of head and neck tumours, when the cannula is removed, the patient should then be encouraged to move his head and neck normally and any postural defect should be corrected by mirror training.

Melanoma of the lower limb may be treated by perfusion similar to that which is used in bypass surgery of the heart. In this case the blood of the affected limb is perfused with the drug of choice; in melanoma this is usually melphalan. Following perfusion the limb is surrounded by ice for 24 hours and any physiotherapy is at the discretion of the surgeon. Normally foot, ankle and quadriceps exercises are allowed at once and gradually increased over two to three days when the patient can start to bear weight and walk. The best results are achieved by teaching partial weight-bearing with crutches until the groin stitches are removed and the wound firmly healed. Then full weight-bearing will be more easily performed. A thorough pre-operative visit by the physiotherapist and strong reassurance that walking will be possible afterwards, is of immense value and greatly to be encouraged.

Chemotherapy is unpleasant for the patient, however well it is supervised, and the physiotherapist must realize this and help in every possible way to ease the discomfort. It really is not possible to state what exactly should be done by way of physical treatment; if a physiotherapist is asked to help in the treatment, then it is essential that she shows herself to be adaptable and resourceful, and she must persevere gently with the patient until the worst is over and improvement and progress is seen. The patient whose condition is deteriorating presents special problems which will be discussed later.

Myeloma

This type of cancer arises from bone marrow cells and is the commonest primary malignant tumour of bone. Whilst many bones may be affected, it can also remain as a solitary deposit. One of the main symptoms is pain and stiffness and a consequent decrease in mobility. Unless the site of the deposit leads to the onset of dramatic symptoms, e.g. paraplegia, these patients can remain undiagnosed for a long while and some indeed will appear in the physiotherapy department under the vague diagnosis of rheumatism or fibrositis.

It is a disease of later years and would appear to be more common in men. Diagnosis may be made on the X-ray appearance of the typical circumscribed areas of bone destruction, or it may be by bone marrow biopsy which enables the myeloma cells to be identified histologically.

The disease is usually treated by drugs but if the lesion is localized it may be treated by radiotherapy. Patients *must* be kept mobile whenever possible. The following case-history describes a typical situation and seeks to show how it was overcome.

CASE-HISTORY

Mrs. L., a housewife of 62, was admitted on 11 February 1969 with a known diagnosis of myeloma. In November 1966 she had been treated for 'rheumatism' of shoulders, arms and neck, with aspirin and bed rest. She had become very inactive. In July 1967, she was admitted to a local hospital with increasing aches and pains; myeloma was diagnosed on X-ray appearance and the bone marrow showed infiltration. She was treated with melphalan and discharged home.

During the following 15 months she became increasingly immobile until finally she was advised to stay in bed. At this point Mrs. L. was told that her condition was incurable and that nothing further could be done. Mrs. L. was not prepared to accept this and with great determination she was able to seek a second opinion in a specialist hospital.

14 February 1969. On admission she was noted to be very frail, though with a determined spirit.

On examination there was gross wasting of all the muscles of the upper limbs, with marked limitation of all shoulder movements, the left being worse than the right. There was gross limitation of all neck movements. Although Mrs. L. was able to feed herself, she had marked limitation of all finger movement, the right being worse than the left, and there was numbness of the first and second fingers of each hand. There was ten degrees of flexion deformity of the knees, due to her having been confined to bed with a pillow under her knees. Mrs. L. also had some difficulty in swallowing.

Programme of treatment. (1) An orthopaedic opinion was sought regarding the hands as it was felt that Mrs. L. had bilateral median nerve compression. This is a complication which may be noted in patients with myeloma and is probably due to the laying down of amyloid deposits.

(2) An aggressive programme of drug therapy was instituted.

(3) Intensive physiotherapy was prescribed with the object of ambulation as quickly as possible.

Physiotherapy. Mrs. L. was treated twice daily with a full table of simple bed exercises for all muscle groups. After the first two days, she was transferred to an orthopaedic hospital for decompression of the median nerves; she was exhorted to maintain the exercises herself.

On her return from hospital, marked improvement was noted in her general condition. Already she was able to move more freely; her joint range had increased by 50 per cent, the numbness of her fingers had gone and she could now hold a newspaper and turn the pages.

She had had no formal physiotherapy whilst in the orthopaedic hospital but had obviously worked extremely hard herself. Among the drugs that she was prescribed, prednisone had undoubtedly helped towards the freer movement.

25 February 1969. Mrs. L. was wheeled to the physiotherapy department and her exercises increased to include slings and springs; walking was commenced between the parallel bars and Mrs. L. herself demanded to try the static bicycle.

Time was also spent with the occupational therapist practising dressing, undressing and household activities.

7 March 1969. Mrs. L. still had ten degrees of flexion contracture at the knee and it was agreed that this should be accepted. It did not appear to restrict her ambulation and her shoes with higher than average heels compensated. Pulleys and ropes were added for shoulder mobilization and a boot and weight of one pound for quadriceps drill.

On the ward, Mrs. L. could usually be found on her bed carrying out her exercises and at the same time advising the other patients to join her!

16 March 1969. Mrs. L. was adjudged independent; she could walk comfortably for 100 yards, climb stairs, dress and undress and feed herself and cut up her own food. She could also make her bed and manage to get in and out of the bath. It was agreed that she should return home and attend the local hospital for maintenance physiotherapy. All drugs were stopped and she was discharged. Arrangements for continuing physiotherapy were initiated before discharge.

May 1969. Mrs. L. was seen in outpatients. She was considerably stiffer and less mobile, and was restarted on prednisone.

June 1969. Greatly improved. Private physiotherapy arrangements excellent. Mrs. L. is able to drive the car, run the house and even do dressmaking.

May 1970. Mrs. L. continued well at home until February 1970 when a course of irradiation was required to relieve pain in her neck. In May 1970 Mrs. L. died from a coronary thrombosis.

Chapter Six: The role of physiotherapy in the treatment of patients receiving radiotherapy

Patients undergoing external irradiation are more likely to require physiotherapy than those who have internal irradiation. However, some patients who may have radioactive gold instilled into the pleura for large effusions may require posturing by the physiotherapists so that the colloidal gold is evenly distributed throughout the pleural cavity. The minimum time should be spent on these occasions. Likewise, gold grains are sometimes implanted into a small circumscribed bladder tumour, or into a carcinoma of head of pancreas. These patients may require urgent chest physiotherapy and again the minimum time should be spent on this treatment.

External irradiation frequently follows surgery, e.g. post-mastectomy, post-laminectomy, post-craniotomy, etc. Sometimes it is done pre-operatively, especially where a patient is elderly or deemed to be a surgical risk and it is hoped that the radiotherapy will bring about a palliation. With sarcomas of bone and soft tissue radiotherapy is used pre-operatively in the hope of preventing spread of cells by the blood during surgery. In other cases, radiotherapy may be given as the treatment of choice, e.g. for a rodent ulcer, for an inoperable cerebral tumour and for a paraplegia which is estimated to have been left too long for a decompression laminectomy to be effective. Some breast cancers may be treated solely by radiotherapy plus hormones, either because the woman will not accept mastectomy, or the tumour is so advanced and fungating that surgery would be dangerous. Radiotherapy is used in the treatment of secondary deposits following breast cancer.

In many cases physiotherapy will be requested at the initial referral; it will be specifically required in all those cases where there is any degree of paralysis. The author is quite dogmatic in her approach to these patients and particularly with the cancer paraplegic: these patients *must* have physiotherapy from the beginning. Many of the most unlikely cases regain almost normal activity and if physiotherapy is withheld until recovery begins, contractures will have developed which may be impossible to release. A patient may thus be disabled when in fact he could have been completely independent. The following case-histories illustrate this.

CASE-HISTORY

Mr. S. was a schoolmaster aged 63 who had shown signs of an incipient paraparesis for some eight weeks before a decompression laminectomy was performed.

12 June 1967. At operation a tumour was found at the level of dorsal 8, and it was noted: 'grey tumour occupying the entire epidural space and surrounding the theca. Tumour exposed to its upper and lower limits and peeled off the theca—immediately the dura began to pulsate. No attempt was made to follow the neoplasm through the intervertebral foramen'. Histological examination showed the tumour to be Hodgkin's disease. The patient was transferred for postoperative irradiation on 22 June 1967.

Note: During this surgical period the patient received no physiotherapy. Ideally, he should have had passive movements to all lower limb joints and encouragement to try and move in bed. General breathing exercises should also be encouraged in these patients.

28 June 1967. Physical examination revealed a frightened, anxious patient whose only wish was to know when he would walk. No active movement could be elicited from the umbilicus downwards. It was noted that already there was some limitation of dorsiflexion of ankle joints, the right being more limited than the left. The upper extremities showed good power.

Observation. It was felt by everyone that recovery of muscle power was extremely doubtful in view of the long history of paraparesis prior to laminectomy. Nevertheless, it was agreed that everything possible should be done so that at worst the patient would be independent in a wheelchair, and at best, if power returned, his joints would be freely mobile to allow full use.

From the beginning, the patient was told quite simply by the physiotherapist that it was not possible to even begin to assess possible recovery, but that everything would be done to ensure his independence within his own physical capabilities. He was encouraged to talk and ask questions and it soon became apparent that sensible explanations went a long way to reassuring him; from the beginning, also, his wife was invited to help in the rehabilitation, even if it only involved making sure that he was consulted about family matters.

Plan of physical treatment. (1) Passive movements to the joints of the lower limbs and stretching of tendo-achilles. Splints were not advised. A cradle and bed board provided a satisfactory support.

(2) General breathing exercises.

(3) General exercises for shoulder girdle and arms, including light springs attached to overhead monkey pole.

Care had to be observed because the laminectomy site was not considered wholly stable. Balance control was not attempted in the early stages.

5 July 1967. Radiotherapy was commenced. It had been decided that the whole spine and para-aortic nodes would be irradiated with the maximum dose to the immediate region of the tumour.

From the commencement of treatment the patient found the radiotherapy extremely trying and great encouragement and reassurance was required at times to even persuade him to continue with it. *Daily* physiotherapy as outlined above was started and this sometimes was repeated twice daily if it was felt that the patient's morale would benefit. It was manifestly clear from the outset that Mr. S. felt that the physiotherapy *was* the most important part of the treatment and consequently his co-operation was ensured and he never failed to send away his visitors if he thought he might otherwise miss his 'exercises'. Stretching of the tendo-achilles was extremely uncomfortable and it required great patience to maintain a reasonable range of dorsiflexion, which remained limited on the right side.

19 July 1967. By this date there was a dramatic improvement in that Mr. S. suddenly found he could flex his knees in bed. Active exercises were now encouraged; simple knee movements were taught with assistance as necessary; static quadriceps contractions were taught, for it was possible to feel a definite contraction.

At the same time it was agreed that sitting over the side of the bed might be attempted. This enabled balance exercises and static holdings to be tried. (It is interesting to note that at no time was Mr. S. *ever* able to sit away from his pillows in long sitting because of pain in his dorsal region and it was deemed advisable not to pursue this.) He was able by means of his monkey pole and minimal help from nurse or physiotherapist to move himself to a position of sitting over the side of the bed. He was taught simple balance exercises and the nurses were invited to help him when they were making his bed. The next step came from the patient himself when he transferred himself from the bed to the commode and with great glee announced this to his physiotherapist. In fact he was invariably one move ahead and this shows all too clearly how important it is to allow the patient to try things out for himself and not always to say: 'No, you are not ready'. It also proves the philosophy of allowing these patients to 'live dangerously'.

26 July 1967. An X-ray on this date showed marked regression of the paravertebral mass and it was agreed that he might sit in a wheelchair. He was taught transfers from bed to chair and back. His arms were extremely strong and he evolved his own particular method of swinging from bed to chair.

Quadriceps power continued to increase and straight leg raising was just possible. Gluteal power was also improving but hip flexion was definitely weak.

16 August 1967. Improvement was now such that Mr. S. was wheeling himself round the hospital and coming daily to the physiotherapy department for more intensive exercise. This included ball games with other patients and as his balance improved the chair arms were removed so that greater effort was required to maintain the upright position. Abdominal and spinal muscles were rapidly improving.

Mr. S. was very anxious to try standing and though he now had control of his knees and hips it was felt he should have a brace to support his dorsal spine. He was therefore fitted for a dorsolumbar brace. (It is the author's experience that braces and calipers are seldom required or indeed justified for cancer paraplegics, but in this case the dorsal spine was adjudged not sufficiently stable to allow walking without the possibility of further collapse of the vertebrae.)

23 August 1967. By now, the radiotherapy had been completed. The brace was awaited and more strenuous exercises were carried out daily including the use of pulleys, springs and weights. A three-pound medicine ball was also used for balance training and throwing, and it is probably true to say that the patient was almost fitter in the upper body than the physiotherapist!

6 September 1967. Excellent control of balance; straight leg raising good. The new brace had arrived and been fitted and the go-ahead was given for standing. This was begun between parallel bars (see Plate 6), and the first two to three days consisted solely of standing and sitting and marking time on the spot. As confidence increased, the first cautious steps were taken, and at the end of ten days Mr. S. would walk easily up and down the parallel bars. At this point consideration was given to the patient's future. Here the greatest help came from Mr. S.'s general practitioner, who not only acted as the go-between of hospital and home but was a tower of strength to everyone who was treating Mr. S. The physiotherapist visited the home with the patient's wife and, apart from the flight of stairs leading to the flat, found no real obstacles to his going home. It was agreed that a second banister should be fixed; also a gate at the top of the stairs, as a safety measure. Loose mats were removed and the flat recarpeted. An entry-phone was installed so that Mr. S. would be able to let in visitors when his wife was out.

Before the physiotherapist assessed the flat, Mr. S. had said to her, 'Don't be put off by the fact that there are stairs. I shall arrange for my friends to carry me up and down until I can manage myself!'

Such was his determination that one was often left feeling utterly inadequate.

By mid-October, Mr. S. was quite independent and ambulant for short distances on a Companion walking frame, and in early November he was discharged home to continue physiotherapy as an outpatient.

December 1967. Mr. S. managed extremely well at home and no problems were encountered. Progression to crutches was accomplished (see Plate 7) and by Christmas Mr. S. was active enough to go with friends not only to church but to a concert as well.

January to April 1968. Progress was rapid over this time despite an attack of shingles affecting the dorsal 8 distribution. Stairs were mastered and an automatic drive car acquired. This latter was converted to hand control (see Plate 8) and a disabled driver's test taken and passed. (In fact his leg power was strong enough to use the foot pedals, but it was felt wise to have hand controls as a precautionary measure.)

Now that Mr. S. was independent and his muscle power considered as strong as possible, he was discharged from attending the physiotherapy department. He continued regular follow-up appointments and steps were taken to find him suitable employment. Again, great help came from the general practitioner who contacted the local education authority where Mr. S. had previously been employed as a teacher. A very suitable post was found for him, coaching educationally backward children.

June 1968. Returned to teaching three mornings a week.

August 1968. Holiday in north Scotland. '... only thing I can't do is jump across moorland streams!'—this was the complaint on a postcard received by the physiotherapist.

September 1968. Working full-time (see Plate 9).

April 1969. Recurrence of disease. Treated May to July with full course of radiotherapy to all remaining gland areas not previously treated.

August 1969. Holiday abroad. Very well.

September 1969. Returned again to full-time teaching.

October 1969 to March 1970. Follow-ups indicated that disease was widespread and Mr. S. was suffering from recurrent bouts of fever. He managed to continue teaching and lead a full life. Chemotherapy started in May 1970.

Taught until end of summer term, then went on holiday to Scotland but had to return because very unwell.

July to October 1970. Slow deterioration interspersed with hospital admissions for transfusions and intensive chemotherapy.

These last three months were a time when courage shone out of both Mr. and Mrs. S.; both realized and understood the situation and there were no difficulties in communication. Mr. S. looked to the physiotherapist to continue to help, and even within 36 hours of his death, he still asked her to help him walk to the sittingroom.

November 1970. Died at home.

This case-history shows clearly how one must never assume anything. From an impossible situation it was possible to follow it through to a marvellous recovery to a life of good quality.

It admirably demonstrates the good rapport between patient and physiotherapist and the value of team discussion.

There were times when it was necessary to get extremely tough with the patient, particularly when he was depressed and miserable during the radiotherapy treatment. Impossible targets were never suggested and, even when recovery looked good, caution was still observed. Care to the point of death was gladly and willingly continued and indeed it would have been quite wrong to have stopped.

CASE-HISTORY

Mr. T. was a business executive aged 46 who had had a right nephrectomy for an adenocarcinoma. Secondary deposits in the lungs had already been noted on the X-rays but no treatment was recommended, the reason for this being that sometimes a spontaneous remission takes place once the primary tumour is removed. Mr. T. made a rapid and uneventful recovery from the operation and returned to work. Three months after this operation he presented with signs and symptoms of cranial disturbance, and on admission to hospital he was conscious though aphasic, and with a complete right hemiplegia. A brain scan showed metastases in both frontal lobes; a chest X-ray showed that the deposits previously noted were progressing.

It was clear that Mr. T. had very advanced disease with a short prognosis. A discussion took place between surgeon and radiotherapist as to the desirability of treatment. The physiotherapist had already been asked to see and treat the patient as necessary.

22 December 1969. On examination the patient was noted to be frightened, apprehensive and aware of everything spoken. The physiotherapist, having introduced herself, explained that she would be seeing him daily to give passive movements to the limbs of his right side and active exercises for the left. His wife was present and so the initial contact was established. Physical examination revealed a total right hemiplegia with some degree of spasticity. The left arm and leg were normal. It had also been agreed that whole brain irradiation should be given and this was also explained to the patient, and indeed the first treatment was given on that day. Plate 10 shows the patient on admission.

24 December 1969. An immediate response was noted; Mr. T. was able to speak slowly though with difficulty in finding words. Some active movement was noted in the gross movement patterns of the arm.

Passive movements were given to the right leg; active assisted movements to the right arm; active exercises to the left leg and arm.

Mr. T. was encouraged to move in bed and to maintain deep breathing exercises. His wife was shown how to help him, particularly allowing him to feed and drink with assistance. The change in Mr. T.'s personality was quite dramatic and his delight was obvious to all. He was treated over the Christmas holiday because it was felt right to maintain his morale. He also continued to receive the irradiation over the holiday.

25 December 1969. Mr. T. celebrated with great aplomb and demonstrated his now adequate use of the right hand by raising his glass to the physiotherapist.

31 December 1969. Mr. T. had good muscular control of his leg and was able to walk to the physiotherapy department for more intensive exercises. From now until his discharge his daily treatment consisted of:

(1) Specific leg exercises emphasizing control and co-ordination.
(2) Bicycling with increasing resistance.
(3) Strengthening of quadriceps muscle with boot and weight.
(4) Increasing walking distance.
(5) Intrinsic finger exercises, e.g. picking up individual marbles and placing them in slotted diathermy felts.
(6) Ball games for balance and co-ordination.

Plate 11 shows Mr. T. on the day of his discharge home.

22 January 1970. Mr. T. was discharged. The only thing he found himself unable to do was to use his electric razor with his right hand. It was felt wiser to encourage him to use the left hand for this, for the chest deposits were rapidly growing, and it was accepted that his life expectancy was very short. It would not be justified to persist in sophisticated techniques.

6 February 1970. Mr. T. died.

Comment. This is a case where physiotherapists and nurses have questioned the rightness of the physical treatment. In defending this, the situation without treatment should be considered. Mr. T. was already helpless and his mental state disturbed whilst he still retained full comprehension. His prognosis did not enter into the discussion; it was felt right that treatment should be given to relieve not only the physical symptoms but the mental distress as well. One of the criteria for active treatment of seemingly terminal patients, is not only the relief of symptoms, mental and physical, but also allowing the patient to die more peacefully and without anguish to the relatives. If Mr. T. had not been treated, he would have become more deeply disturbed and distressed because he could neither move nor communicate. His family would have suffered untold agonies through having to watch a deteriorating situation and being helpless to act.

From a nursing point of view, catheterization, etc., would have been necessary, together with all the care for a heavy paralysed patient. For the physiotherapist, an ever-increasing problem of facing a patient undergoing no improvement. Thus, for every reason, treatment for such a patient was absolutely right and his last three weeks were spent in complete happiness with his family at home.

CASE-HISTORY

Mr. E. was an engineer aged 49 who in November 1969 underwent a laminectomy for the removal of an ependymoma involving the lower end of the spinal cord. Following operation he received a full course of irradiation to the whole brain and spinal cord. In July 1970 he had to undergo further decompression laminectomy because of a recurrence leading to increasing pain and weakness of his legs. In October 1970 he was started on intermittent courses of vincristine with some improvement of his condition. In March 1971 he was admitted for general nursing care and assessment of his physical condition.

23 March 1971. On admission he was assessed by the nurses as being difficult and unco-operative, but this was never apparent to the physiotherapists! Physical examination revealed good power in the quadriceps and gluteal muscles but some weakness of the anterior tibial muscles with resultant foot drop. Co-ordination of movements of the lower limbs was very poor, and there was virtually no feeling in the soles of the feet with consequent loss of positioning sense. (Vincristine is a known neurotoxic and was probably a contributory factor to these obvious neurological signs.)

Mr. E. was only able to walk on crutches with the maximum help of two people. He was able to sit for only short periods in a chair because of pain in his lower back.

Direct questioning revealed that he had first complained of back pain in 1966, for which he had received 'pills'. In 1968, the pain had increased to such an extent that he was finally admitted for investigation, and not until November 1969 was a decompression laminectomy performed.

Mr. E. was married, but his wife was an inadequate personality who was at this time quite incapable of accepting the situation and indeed was the direct cause of Mr. E.'s admission. She had been led to understand that he was likely 'to sever the spinal cord and to become totally paralysed'. For this reason she decided she would never be able to cope and that the best thing was to arrange for admission of her husband to a 'terminal' home. This was the situation which presented itself to the physiotherapists.

Aims of treatment. (1) To improve co-ordination of movement of the lower limbs.

(2) To mobilize on elbow crutches.

(3) To make as independent as possible within his own limitations.

(4) To help the wife accept the situation and enable the patient to return home.

From the commencement of treatment there was never any doubt about the enthusiasm of the patient and his willing cooperation for really intensive work was remarkable.

Plan of treatment. (1) Mr. E. took part in all general classwork and activities with the other patients. This had the dual object of using all muscles as well as helping him to become acclimatized to sitting for longer periods at a time.

(2) He was taught Frenkel's exercises; patterns were permanently marked out on the floor and he was thus able to take himself off to practise many times during the day. Whenever he found that sitting in a chair was becoming too tiring and painful, he would transfer himself to a plinth for a rest.

(3) Walking training was commenced between the parallel bars and progressed to using elbow crutches with a four-point gait.

26 April 1971. Marked improvement in co-ordination and control of feet. Mr. E. still had no sensation in the feet and walked with eyes down and a broad base. He was quite independent in mobility with the exception of stairs. The question was now raised about returning home.

19 May 1971. Mr. E.'s progress had been well maintained and it was agreed that discharge home was the right move. He was able to be downstairs and so the question of stairs did not arise. Full social services were arranged. Arrangements were also made to re-admit him again after one month to re-assess the situation. His wife made no attempt to keep any appointments made in order to discuss his condition; she accepted his discharge.

21 May 1971. Mr. E. was discharged.

21 June 1971. Mr. E. was re-admitted for re-assessment. Physical examination revealed *no* deterioration and his walking with crutches was much improved. The patient admitted that his wife was extremely unhelpful and was virtually out all day.

It was agreed that he should have a further month's intensive rehabilitation with the emphasis again on co-ordination exercises and that progression to negotiating stairs be attempted. At the same time it was agreed that his wife must be seen by the physiotherapist so that his condition could be explained to her. In particular it was necessary that she be given to understand just how much Mr. E. could do and how much help he would require.

28 June 1971. Mrs. E. was seen. She proved to be most unhelpful; it was gently explained to her that she would have to learn to make allowances for her husband's 'difficult temperament', as she put it, and that this was partly due to the frustrations resultant from the disease. She was shown how best to help him when necessary and was assured that if insuperable problems arose, he would always be re-admitted and that, in any case, he could return for periodic intensive rehabilitation.

6 July 1971. Mr. E. was discharged home, this time able to manage stairs. The local authority social services department arranged for additional banisters as necessary, as well as 'grab rails' in the bathroom and lavatory. They also ramped two shallow steps from the garden to street level.

December 1971. A home visit was paid. Mr. E. had greatly improved. He was attending the local hospital for maintenance physiotherapy twice weekly and had arranged to return to work also for two afternoons per week. His employer arranged the transport for this. There was no sign of his wife and Mr. E. stated that she 'gave him no confidence'. He himself was clearly well; he was managing stairs and continuing with intermittent courses of vincristine.

June 1973. Mr. E. was re-admitted for a short period of rehabilitation whilst his wife was on holiday.

On examination (consultant's comment): 'Very well. Has put on two stone in weight. Walking easily with elbow crutches—aching pain in legs all day. Has been provided with an invalid car. He is still working two afternoons a week and takes himself there in his car. He has obviously mellowed in outlook since last seen 18 months ago.'

It was agreed that he should progress from crutches to sticks and that he should be given a strict diet to help control and reduce his weight.

Perhaps the most interesting part of this re-admission was the meeting with Mrs. E. The change in this lady was remarkable to behold; she could now accept the situation and was unquestionably a great support to her husband. Her words expressed everything. 'I realize that my husband and I are in this together and that I must help him.' From the physiotherapist's point of view it was doubly gratifying. Here was a so-called 'terminal' patient still enjoying life and a dubious marriage relationship now firmly established on mutual understanding.

With this type of patient where brain and spinal tumours or secondary deposits are being treated either by radiotherapy alone or by radiotherapy combined with another form of treatment, the prognosis will be varied. If it is short, every effort should be made to get the patient as independent as possible in order that he may go home, even though it may only be for a short time. Precise treatments should not be attempted, and the relatives should be encouraged to allow the patient to do as much as possible for himself.

When the prognosis is reasonably hopeful, more time may be spent on specific treatments, and if the tumour has been effectively removed before permanent brain or spinal cord damage has occurred, good recovery of function can be expected. In patients who receive radiotherapy for a brain tumour which is unsuitable for surgery, recovery will be variable depending on how effectively the tumour can be destroyed without damage to normal brain tissue.

In patients who have brain tumours or cerebral deposits, the intelligence more often than not remains unimpaired. This must be remembered, particularly when speech or sight is impaired. Patience has to be exercised in listening to such patients trying to express themselves, for they become very frustrated and do not like being hurried. Patients who are treated with irradiation for a brain tumour will lose their hair (epilation). Wigs must be available for them *at once* and not ordered after the hair has fallen out. A great deal of understanding of this problem is required, and reassurance given to the patient so that he or she understands that the hair will grow again.

Chapter Seven: **Rehabilitation for patients with breast cancer**

Cancer of the breast causes over 10,000 deaths annually in England and Wales, and each year many thousands of women undergo mastectomy. This is essentially a female problem, but a very small number of men also undergo mastectomy annually. It is not proposed, however, to discuss them.

To a woman, the breast emphasizes her essential femininity and as a consequence emotional influences are very strong. The initial findings of a lump in the breast can, in some cases, cause sheer panic. It is so important for women to realize that only a very small proportion of lumps are of significance, and everything possible should be done to encourage them to seek advice at the earliest time. From the very beginning of the investigation of a breast lump, the patient must feel that everyone is supporting her, including her husband (if married), her family, the general practitioner and the hospital staff. Confidence at this stage will do much to enable the patient to face the future with equanimity.

Mastectomy

The operation may be of several types.

RADICAL MASTECTOMY

This is the traditional Halsted operation which entails removal of the whole breast together with the pectoral major and minor muscles and the axillary lymph nodes. The incision used to extend from the xiphisternum, over the shoulder and into the upper arm; nowadays skilled and sympathetic surgeons will use an incision from the tip of the coracoid process to the xiphisternum. Thus it is possible for women to wear sleeveless dresses, and the formation of a string-like adhesion across the axilla is avoided. Plate 12 shows the incision of a carefully sited radical mastectomy.

MODIFIED RADICAL MASTECTOMY

This is a variety of the true radical, sometimes known as the Patey mastectomy. The whole breast is removed, but the pectoral muscles are conserved and only the upper axillary nodes can be removed.

SIMPLE MASTECTOMY

In this case only the breast tissue is removed.

Within these three main types will be found many refinements. Sometimes only a wedge resection will be performed. A great deal of discussion is continuing today as to the relative values of these operations, and whilst this does not directly concern the physiotherapist, it is of additional interest to study the different types, and to note the way in which the patients progress afterwards. The type of operation used may also be dependent on the staging of the disease. For example, some surgeons will always advocate radical mastectomy for stages 1 and 2 as the best chance of eradicating the disease, whereas stages 3 and 4 would be treated by radiotherapy initially and might be followed by a simple mastectomy for the stage 3. Every surgeon will have different views; already there have been a number of controlled trials whose final results appear to be equivocal, although it would seem that radical mastectomy is still the operation which carries the greater survival rate (Atkins, Hayward, Klugner & Wayte, 1972).

Physiotherapy following breast cancer

Whatever type of operation is performed, the physiotherapist must apprise herself of the surgeon's wishes as to how much exercise he will allow. In no other field of surgical practice is there so much indecision regarding the place of the physiotherapist, and one should be cautious of the surgeon who says 'Do what you like'. Injudicious physiotherapy can lead to delayed healing, capsulitis of the shoulder and swelling of the arm. The variety of instructions given will include 'No shoulder movement for seven days with the arm bandaged to the side' and 'Full shoulder elevation and rotation on the day following operation'. There is no doubt that full elevation at once can lead to acute capsulitis of the shoulder and this can be very intractable to treat. Arms bandaged to the side of the body seldom lead to stiff shoulders and where there is some restriction of elevation this will soon come out with pendulum swinging exercises.

In no circumstances whatsoever should passive or forced elevation be carried out.

Physiotherapy for patients following a simple mastectomy is rarely required, but if it is, the same principles will apply.

Suggested pattern of treatment for a patient following radical mastectomy

PRE-OPERATIVE

The physiotherapist should introduce herself to the patient and explain carefully what will be required of her after the operation. She must be prepared to discuss prostheses and any other problem which may be worrying her. It will probably be worthwhile to offer to sort out problems, for patients are often reluctant to discuss trifling matters with busy surgeons, and yet though they may be simple to resolve, to a patient quite trifling things can appear mountainous. The establishment beforehand of this easy relation-

ship will show the patient that she can expect similar help
wards. The nursing staff will be equally involved with this ge.
reassurance and the physiotherapist should be willing to share
discussions with the nurses where it concerns them.

The amount of movement that will be possible postoperatively will depend on the surgeon's instructions and should be explained to the patient. In all cases the patient may use her hand and lower arm. (One hopes that the intravenous drip will not be inserted into the arm of the mastectomy side.)

Breathing exercises should be taught, particularly lower, lateral costal breathing. The patient will probably have a firm crêpe bandage round the chest to secure the dressing and to control fluid formation under the flaps, and consequently she may not breathe as deeply as she should.

The necessity for as much movement as possible in bed, and particularly the need to carry out definite leg exercises, should be explained. There is no need to mention the word 'thrombosis'; it is easier to talk about moving the legs to prevent them aching. Patients are invariably up within 24 hours and able to move around freely. They should also be reassured that they will have a drainage bottle that can be safely carried around or put in the dressing-gown pocket; and that it will not prevent them from walking about.

POSTOPERATIVE

Day 1. Be prepared to find a depressed patient, for quite often they do feel miserable.

Lateral costal breathing exercises should be checked and one should be certain that the chest is clear.

Leg exercises and general position in bed should be checked.

In *all* cases hand clenching and stretching, finger flexion, wrist flexion and extension, supination and pronation should be checked. If the arm is bandaged to the side, shoulder shrugging and static deltoid contractions should be encouraged.

If elevation is required, the weight of the arm should be taken and the patient asked to raise her arm above her head.

Days 2 to 7, or until drains are removed. The patient will be freely mobile as soon as the intravenous drip is down.

Check posture and make quite certain that the patient is standing correctly, with shoulders level and weight evenly distributed.

Check arm movements as required.

Encourage normal activities as much as possible.

If a prosthesis has been provided, there is absolutely no reason why this should not be worn, in fact it should be encouraged. If the patient wishes to get dressed this also should be encouraged, though it may not be very practicable until the drains are removed.

After the drains are removed. Full active exercises may now be encouraged. *Forced* movements must never be carried out. Abduction of the shoulder should be carried out carefully until the flaps are firmly adherent to the chest wall. If abduction is performed too early or too vigorously, fluid will collect under the flaps which will need to be aspirated regularly. This is not to be desired; no patient likes a needle being inserted unless essential and also each time a needle is used there is always a small risk of infection.

Pendulum swinging exercises are to be encouraged. The patient is seated on a stool with the affected arm hanging free, the body leaning forward and the arm allowed to hang heavily and swing in a sagittal plane impelled by its own weight. This can be repeated, swinging across the body in a transverse plane. As the movement improves, the patient can progress to performing the exercises from standing.

Arm circling may also be taught, from an elbow bend position.

It cannot be overstressed, however, that normal activities are really the best form of movement for any patient after mastectomy. These should include eating, drinking, washing, doing one's hair, dressing, etc. Reassurance all through treatments that full movements will be achieved is the keynote to success.

Most patients are discharged at ten to fourteen days after operation, and by then they should have practically full movement. If they are to have a postoperative course of radiotherapy, it is advisable to see them as outpatients to check that movement is maintained. Sometimes post-mastectomy radiation leads to skin reaction, and the consequent soreness and skin tightening leads to patients being reluctant to move.

On discharge, patients should be advised about future management. The Marie Curie Memorial Foundation issues a leaflet especially for patients who have undergone mastectomy. The following is an extract from its 'do's and don'ts':

> 'For your own sake do be careful when carrying out the following activities:
>
> (1) Lifting heavy articles from the floor.
>
> (2) Reaching upwards for heavy saucepans, tins, boxes, etc.
>
> (3) Carrying shopping baskets, heavy handbags, etc., on the affected side.
>
> (4) Digging the garden and over-use of the arm.
>
> (5) If there is marked arm swelling, be careful to avoid minor injuries of the skin such as scratches, etc. When pruning roses in particular and gardening in general, *always* wear leather gloves. It is possible to cause an infection if this advice is not accepted. For the same reason, care should be taken when manicuring, particularly the cuticles.
>
> (6) When sunbathing, and particularly if radiotherapy has been given, care should be taken not to allow too much sun on the affected side. A silk or cotton scarf may be thrown over the arm to prevent this occurring.
>
> In all the above instances let commonsense and moderation guide you, but when in doubt, ask someone to help you!'

All patients should have it explained to them that regular follow-up appointments are absolutely essential. These will probably be monthly in the first instance, then gradually lengthening as the time after the operation increases.

Many women after mastectomy never have any further trouble; they adapt themselves and their lives to the situation. Husbands can be of great support to their wives in encouraging them and by appearing not revolted by the fact that a breast has been amputated. Sexual problems may require advice in a minority of cases and they should be dealt with sympathetically by expert counsellors. Clothing problems should likewise be dealt with swiftly. It should be possible for all mastectomy patients to wear the clothes they wore before their operation. In fact, the last thing they should do is to wear unusual clothes as this only draws attention to themselves.

The physiotherapist can offer tactful and reassuring advice and if she cannot help she must be prepared to go and find someone who can. She should have some knowledge of the type of prostheses available, but again, personal likes will dictate in the end what best suits the individual patient. The main types available in this country are the granule-filled, the oil-filled and the silicone gel type. What matters most is the weight content: the prosthesis must match the remaining breast in weight, as otherwise the patient will suffer strain on the dorsal spine and consequently develop a postural defect. Most patients prefer to wear the brassière that they have always worn and insert the prosthesis into a pocket sewn into the brassière cup. Care must be taken that the pocket will allow the tail of the prosthesis to fall round the lateral aspect of the chest wall. Plate 13 shows a patient following radical mastectomy with her prosthesis in position.

Additional surgical procedures for patients with breast cancer

Whereas many women have their cancer confined to the breast and live many years of good life, others develop secondary deposits (metastases). Metastases from breast cancer are usually found in bone, and consequently the physiotherapist will be deeply involved. Some breast cancers are hormone-dependent, and the first surgical procedure contemplated after the onset of deposits is bilateral oophorectomy with local radiotherapy.

Indeed, because of this known dependency, some surgeons will do a routine bilateral oophorectomy at the time of the initial mastectomy, particularly if the patient is under 50 and has already had a family.

Oophorectomy as such is straightforward and seldom requires

a great deal of help from the physiotherapist. If, however, the deposits are in the pelvis or lower limbs then bed exercises and graduated active mobilization will be necessary.

If the patient is post-menopausal and under 65, bilateral adrenalectomy is usually performed. This is done through the abdomen, involving opening the peritoneum, or alternatively, laterally through the bed of each twelfth rib. In both cases, but particularly if the second method is adopted, deep breathing exercises are essential. The pleura is easily nicked when excising a rib, and a pneumothorax is a not uncommon complication. Should the ribs themselves be affected by deposits, care must be exercised with vibrations and shakings.

Quite dramatic results can follow these operations, allowing the patient up to five or more years of good life. One must be philosophical about these operations. Usually patients are told exactly what the chances of success are and they are usually willing to accept the gamble. Approximately 50 per cent of adrenalectomies are successful and the length of good life may be one to ten years.

Replacement therapy in the form of cortisone has to be given, and the patient remains on the drug for the rest of her life. She must be fully aware of the need to take her medicine regularly and if she feels ill to report at once to her doctor. All patients on steroids should carry a card with them giving the dosage. If a hypophysectomy (removal of the pituitary gland) is carried out, then the replacement therapy will also include pitressin and thyroid extract.

CASE-HISTORY

Mrs. B. was a housewife of 42 who was seen in a breast clinic with a lump in the right breast which she stated had been present for one week. On examination there was a 3 × 5 cm hard mobile mass in the upper inner quadrant with a firm mobile node palpable in the right axilla. Mammography examination was negative, but thermography positive. She was admitted for biopsy of the lump, which was found to be a scirrhous carcinoma. It was decided to treat her with irradiation. After the course was completed Mrs. B. attended as an outpatient and for six months was very well.

December 1967. Mrs. B. complained of 'fibrositis' of the neck, hips and legs, and X-rays showed secondary deposits in the pelvis. It was decided to treat her with hormones, in this case Durabolin. For a further six months she remained well.

July 1968. Mrs. B. complained of increasing pain in her lower lumbar spine and pelvis, and it was decided to give her a course of irradiation. She then remained consistently well for a further 12 months. She also received prednisone during this time.

September 1969. Mrs. B. was admitted for a course of irradiation to her cervical spine. She was in considerable pain and the X-rays showed marked destruction of the third, fourth and fifth cervical vertebral bodies. A collar was requested. This was the first time that a physiotherapist had been involved in Mrs. B.'s treatment, and on first acquaintance she was frightened, in pain, and clearly apprehensive of everybody and everything. A firm adjustable Zimmer collar was fitted with some difficulty, but once Mrs. B. appreciated the relief of pain, she agreed happily to wear it. It is doubtful whether the relief of pain was because of the collar but this was not a time to disagree with the patient! The collar was necessary to prevent collapse of the bodies of the vertebrae whilst consolidation took place after the irradiation.

October 1969. Mrs. B. was discharged home.

15 December 1969. Mrs. B. was admitted with very acute pain in her pelvis. It was felt that this was a 'terminal' admission. The X-rays showed multiple deposits throughout the pelvis, with fractures of the pubic rami and dangerously sited deposits in the medullae of both femora with a particularly dangerous one in the left femur extending to the cortex. She was quite unable to do anything.

18 December 1969. Her pain was rapidly controlled by suitably prescribed medication and, though very ill, she was alert to the situation and was not prepared to accept lying in bed.

The physiotherapist was asked to give bed exercises. Mrs. B. was never an easy patient, particularly at this stage; she exhibited all the reactions of denial, rejection and annoyance and all the physiotherapists concerned came in for a share of the abuse! (This was a case where it was decided to share her care equally between all members of the department. Normally it is obviously better for one physiotherapist to treat a patient all the time.)

Over Christmas, Mrs. B. lapsed into a coma and all active treatment including physiotherapy was withdrawn. After a period of three to four weeks she rallied, and began demanding exercises and even to be allowed to get out of bed. Physiotherapy was restarted and it was gently explained that her legs were too brittle to allow her to stand or get out of bed, but that she would be given some medicine to help them. She was given thiotepa, one of the drugs used in disseminated breast cancer. The physiotherapist found that by explaining to Mrs. B. that the exercises were necessary to help her to become sufficiently strong to get out of bed, full co-operation and understanding was finally reached. Physiotherapy was then accepted. Exercises could only consist of active exercises to all muscle groups of the lower limbs with particular emphasis on static quadriceps contractions. There was a very real danger of fracture and resisted exercises were not possible. In spite of such limitations Mrs. B.'s muscle power did improve considerably and straight leg raising was just possible.

May 1970. Mrs. B. was so much better in herself and yet so bitterly frustrated at being confined to bed that the consultant decided to offer her the option of a bilateral adrenalectomy. This she accepted gladly, in the full knowledge that it might be unsuccessful. The X-rays at this time still showed gross deposits throughout the pelvis.

9 June 1970. Bilateral adrenalectomy was performed and Mrs. B. made an uneventful recovery. Her leg exercises were increased and it was agreed that some manual resistance might be added. This was achieved with no ill-effects and the use of light springs with sling support was substituted. This was set up in the ward using the overhead bed handle, and Mrs. B. was able to spend a long time each day doing her exercises. Short periods many times a day was felt to be safer than a long period once or twice a day.

7 July 1970. Although the X-rays showed no appreciable change, Mrs. B. was now moving freely round the bed; she could 'straight leg raise' comfortably, and her quadriceps muscle power was good. It was decided that this was the moment that walking with partial weight-bearing might be permitted. The consultant explained to the patient that there might be a risk of fracture but he felt this was minimal and that it was a justifiable risk. The physiotherapist also explained this very thoroughly to Mrs. B. and told her quite simply that not only were the bones still 'brittle and moth-eaten' but that she herself was not a light weight! Mrs. B. was, by now, extremely grateful and sensible about the situation and fully accepted it by saying, 'I can't stay in bed all the time. Let's get on with it and see what happens.'

Walking was started between the parallel bars and rapidly progressed to elbow crutches. Mrs. B. had no pain in her pelvis or legs and was rapidly mobilised.

23 July 1970. Mrs. B. was discharged home and within six weeks had returned to the part-time job that she had had when first taken ill.

This case admirably demonstrates the gloriously unexpected result as well as the need to take the calculated risk despite the X-ray appearance.

Hypophysectomy, removal of the pituitary gland, is yet another operation sometimes performed instead of oophorectomy and adrenalectomy. It is performed through a trans-sphenoidal incision, and because the patient is usually nursed recumbent afterwards, physiotherapy by way of breathing exercises and leg exercises will be required. Sometimes, if the deposits are extensive in the spine, the patient may be in a spinal jacket and physiotherapy will be even more vital.

If surgical removal of these ductless glands is deemed unwise, a similar result may be obtained by:

(1) giving radiotherapy to the ovaries and thus inducing a radiation menopause;

(2) giving cortisone as a medication and thereby inducing a medical adrenalectomy;

(3) implanting yttrium rods in the pituitary fossa and producing a radiation ablation.

As has been stated, when the breast tumour is hormone-dependent, striking results will be obtained. When these measures fail, it is still possible to offer palliation by means of irradiation or chemotherapy or a combination of both.

At this point it is right to stress that limbs which have been affected with bone deposits may be handled without fear, provided it is done with firmness and sympathy. The patient will sense at once whether the physiotherapist or nurse is frightened and this fear will be transmitted. Always reassure the patient before handling a limb, and if pain is known to result from handling, then advise the patient first.

Always look at X-rays to see where the deposits are situated. If the patient is to walk, this latter fact is important.

(1) If a deposit lies in the medulla of the shaft of the femur, it is safe to walk.

(2) If a deposit is in the cortex, but with some clearance from the edge, the patient may walk, but with caution and probably with two crutches rather than one stick.

(3) If a deposit is in the cortex and right at the edge, non-weight bearing may be allowed if the patient is heavy, or partial weight-bearing if light, with two crutches may be allowed. If both legs are affected, walking should not be undertaken until the deposits have healed or sclerosed.

It is an interesting fact that a femur or pelvis, which gives the impression on X-ray of being completely moth-eaten, may still be extremely strong. If the deposits are in the pubic rami, the anterior portion of the ilium or crest of the ilium, there is no danger in walking, as these are non-weight-bearing areas. Great care should be observed if the deposits are in close proximity to the acetabulum as there may be a risk of central fracture and dislocation of the hip.

Deposits in the cervical spine almost always require the patient to be fitted with a collar, either soft or rigid depending on the extent and precise position of the deposit. Deposits in the dorsal or lumbar spine may require either a brace or a corset, again depending on the position and symptoms. Surgical appliances should only be advised where they are absolutely necessary for the wellbeing of the patient. As has been said, many of these deposits, although looking horrid, are in fact quite strong, and it is quite wrong to inflict a greater burden on the patient by ordering complicated braces and splints. As the majority of these patients are women, a decent well-fitting corset from a department store may well be more acceptable than a complicated surgical appliance with numerous belts and buckles.

Lymphoedema

One of the complications which may follow radical mastectomy is lymphoedema. This is in part due to the removal of the axillary lymph nodes, but it may also be due to thrombosis of the axillary vein, either at the time of operation or postoperatively through forced stretching of the arm. It also appears to follow more often when radiotherapy is given postoperatively.

Most patients will develop a minimal oedema that will settle itself or remain the same for many years. For those who develop a greater degree of oedema, the following physiotherapeutic treatments may help. At present there is no evidence that any one treatment is better than another, and what will help one patient may have quite the reverse effect on another.

(1) Deep massage in elevation with hand and finger exercises. The arm should be placed in elevation, supported fully on pillows. The massage should commence at the proximal point and gradually move distally down the limb. Deep effleurage and kneading will be the massage of choice. The massage should be followed by intensive active finger and hand exercises.

(2) Faradism under pressure in elevation, with the electrodes bandaged in position by means of a rubber bandage or an elastic webbing bandage. This bandage should extend the whole length of the arm from metacarpal heads to upper arm.

(3) Sinusoidal stimulation in elevation. (This is a treatment which is probably not carried out nowadays.)

(4) The Jobst compression unit.

JOBST COMPRESSION UNIT

This is a form of treatment which originated in the United States.

The apparatus. The machine is a light-weight pneumatic pump, weighing approximately 15 pounds, which is designed to provide intermittent pneumatic compression. The period of compression can be regulated as can the pressure control. The control panel consists of an *on-off* switch, an indicator lamp, a pressure control valve, an *on* timer control, an *off* timer control and a pressure outlet stem. The pumping mechanism is connected by rubber tubing to a double-layered, sealed, plastic sheath, which is made of Neoprene impregnated nylon (see Plate 14).

Method of treatment. The patient is treated on a bed with the arm fully supported on pillows (see Plate 15), or in an easy chair with the arm supported. The patient should indicate in which position she is most comfortable; this is a particularly important thing to achieve since the treatment takes a minimum of $1\frac{1}{2}$ hours on each visit. The treatment programme should be explained to the patient before the actual start. Co-operation is of great importance and time spend on adequate explanations will always be repaid many times.

The arm is bared and the shoulder straps slipped down; all rings are removed including where necessary and if possible the wedding ring. Watches and bracelets are also removed. The arm is encased in Tubegauz (size 78) before being placed in the compression sleeve. (A sleeve of some form of cotton material is essential since the arm will sweat very considerably in the nylon sheath and will become rather soggy.) The rubber tubing is then attached both to the machine and the sleeve; the machine is switched on and the sleeve inflated to the required pressure. It should always be possible for the patient to wriggle her fingers inside the inflated sleeve. The control switches are normally set in a ratio of 3:1, i.e. 45 seconds compression and 15 seconds off. The pressure is adjusted to between 45 and 60 mm Hg, according to the patient's tolerance.

Treatment duration. The duration of treatment for each patient is dependent on the patient's tolerance and acceptance of the treatment and the ease with which the patient can attend for treatment.

Contra-indications. The Jobst compression unit must not be used where there is any evidence of cellulitis or reddening of the skin. If there is any pain or discomfort during the treatment, the machine should be turned off and the treatment discontinued.

After-treatment. Following treatment patients should carry out hand exercises, i.e. finger flexion and extension, wrist flexion and extension, and wrist circling. These should be carried out as often as possible at home with the arm in elevation supported on pillows. Patients should also be advised to posture the arm at night and whenever they are sitting down. The lifting of heavy weights should be discouraged, likewise forced upward elevation of the shoulder.

Plates 16 and 17 show a lymphoedematous arm before and after treatment by the Jobst Unit.

ELASTIC SLEEVES

The value of wearing elastic sleeves is debatable and some surgeons do not like them because of the additional constriction of the upper part of the arm. If they are used, they should be put on immediately on rising and should be so designed as to come over the shoulder and right down to the heads of the metacarpals. A double thickness of the appropriate width of Tubigrip with a hole cut for the thumb, is a very adequate night support or for wearing round the house and garden. A heavy seamless stretch nylon stocking with the foot cut off, makes an extremely good sleeve. The lower cut end should just be folded in and it can be safely secured by wearing a wristwatch. The upper edge should be left free and this avoids the tight band which often leads to constriction of the upper arm. Many women dislike wearing special sleeves as it draws attention to their disability.

Sometimes the lymphoedema can reach such proportions and

cause such severe disability that the only practical solution is disarticulation at the shoulder joint. It is always hoped that adequate physiotherapy treatments may at least keep the oedema in proportion and enable the patient to fulfil her activities. The weight of the oedema may be such as to cause a traction palsy of the brachial plexus. Supporting the arm in a sling may help to relieve this and movements of the fingers and hand should be encouraged.

Chapter Eight: **Rehabilitation for patients undergoing head and neck surgery**

Within this branch of surgery dramatic advances have been made possible by improved anaesthesia and postoperative care. Many cancers around the jaw and mouth are considered curable if treated early and by radical surgery. Much of this surgery is of a mutilating kind and requires a great deal of reconstruction; the physiotherapist can be involved in treating such patients over many months.

The prospect of mutilation will lead to patients feeling sensitive about their appearance, and rehabilitation will be two-fold in approach:

(1) Purely local treatment by physiotherapeutic means.

(2) Reorientation into society, so that the patient may feel confident to mix with others and return to work where possible.

It is the second of these approaches that will make or mar the success of the surgeon. For what purpose is there, if having removed the tumour successfully, the patient becomes a hermit and society ostracizes him?

General principles for all head and neck patients

PRE-OPERATIVE CARE

It is hoped, and it will be assumed, that the physiotherapist is regarded as part of the team looking after these patients, and in consequence she will see pre-operatively all patients who are to undergo major surgery. A speech therapist should be available for such patients also, and the physiotherapist can often offer useful help to her by the teaching of good breathing exercises for laryngectomy patients and in carrying out mouth exercises for some patients who have tongue surgery.

The physiotherapist should introduce herself to the patient and explain simply and clearly what her part is in the treatment plan and what will be required from the patient. If there is to be extensive surgery the patient requires reassurance from everybody that everything will be done to ensure that the end result will not lead to incapacitation.

Teach breathing exercises, lower lateral costal and diaphragmatic. If there is to be a tracheostomy, and this is common practice as a temporary measure, explain how a nurse will suck out the secretions whilst the physiotherapist vibrates the chest.

Check the range of movement of neck and shoulders. This is important to know pre-operatively, since patients are reluctant to move their necks afterwards and may get quite stiff.

Teach shoulder shrugging exercises. If a block dissection of the cervical lymph nodes is to be carried out, the spinal accessory nerve will almost certainly be sacrificed and consequently the trapezius muscle will be partly denervated.

Teach mouth and jaw exercises if a mandibulectomy or glossectomy is considered. The judicious use of a mirror may help but some patients are self-conscious and may not appreciate having to look at themselves.

Teach posture correction and explain the need to move around in bed as much as possible afterwards. Most of these patients are able to sit out of bed quite soon. If surgery is on the cervical oesophagus with replacement, it may be necessary to fix the neck in partial flexion for a few days to avoid strain on the graft, and this should be explained to the patient. The physiotherapist may indeed be asked to provide the splint to hold the neck in flexion. This can be achieved by making a light plaster or polythene splint and holding it in position with a forehead strap and shoulder straps.

Be prepared to answer and explain all kinds of questions which the patient may ask. The consultant will have explained the operative procedure but it is the finer points which the patient often wants clarified, and this is again where the physiotherapist can help. This does not minimize in any way the part which the nursing staff will also play, but experience has shown that a good rapport between surgeon and physiotherapist can be of priceless value.

POSTOPERATIVE CARE

It is not intended to describe operative procedures in detail but physiotherapists will appreciate the situation much better if they can watch some of these operations and see for themselves exactly what is carried out.

Normally patients who undergo head and neck surgery will be up within 24 to 48 hours and it is interesting to observe that patients who undergo very extensive procedures do not appear to suffer a great deal of pain; discomfort may be felt but this is controllable by simple analgesics. Reassurance is necessary where movement is concerned so that patients do not become afraid of damaging themselves. All patients who undergo this type of surgery will benefit from massage to the shoulder girdle. Muscle spasm will be relieved and the general circulation to the area stimulated.

BLOCK DISSECTION OF CERVICAL LYMPH NODES

This operation is frequently carried out either in isolation or as part of a major procedure. The spinal accessory nerve which lies close to the superficial cervical lymph glands is almost always sacrificed. If shoulder shrugging exercises are taught and insisted upon from the commencement, there should be no difficulty in maintaining good tone in the trapezius muscle. If, however, this is not carried out the patient may be left with atrophied trapezii, drooping shoulders and consequent pressure on the nerve roots leading to acroparaesthesia and weakness of the hands.

Laryngectomy

Patients who develop cancer of the larynx are usually treated initially with irradiation. This is to preserve the voice. Occasionally if the cancer is confined very locally to one cord, a partial excision of the vocal cord may be performed, but this is not generally advocated. Patients undergoing radiotherapy for laryngeal cancer seldom require physiotherapy unless they develop a chest infection, when general chest physiotherapy would be given. If the patient is elderly or if there is a degree of stridor then the treatment must be graded accordingly. Occasionally the larynx and glottis can become severely oedematous so that emergency tracheostomy is necessary, and physiotherapy requested. In this instance the patient is usually very frightened and apprehensive and extra patience and reassurance is required. Relaxation and controlled breathing can go a long way to relieving this distress.

When laryngectomy is performed the general principles already outlined apply. Though the voice box is removed the patient is not deaf. One so often comes across nurses and others shouting at patients following laryngectomy (Tait, 1971). For the first seven to ten days laryngectomy patients must not attempt to make any sound; they should be encouraged to mouth their words for this also acts as practical exercise for the muscles of phonation. They should be supplied with a writing pad and pen or pencil, or better still with a magic writer. When conversing with these patients it is kinder to word one's questions so that a shake or nod of the head is all that is required for an answer.

Good controlled breathing exercises will not only help the patient's chest but will help the speech therapist when she comes to begin to teach him to speak again by means of oesophageal speech. Immense patience is required on the part of the patient as well as great encouragement from all members of the team and the family and friends. It is so easy to say, 'Write it down', rather than finding time to sit down and allow the patient to speak slowly. Patients vary considerably in their aptitude to learn to speak, and much of the success or failure depends on the degree of rapport and confidence which is established between the patient and the therapists. If a patient fails to learn to speak he can use an electronic vibrator which does at least enable him to communicate, though in a very monotonous voice.

Some trials are being undertaken on the efficacy of implanting mechanical voice boxes, but there is no satisfactory breakthrough yet. Much of this work has been done in the United States, but it is felt that if patients are not capable of learning to produce an oesophageal voice then it is extremely unlikely that they can learn to cope with the implanted device. Shedd *et al.* (1972) describe one of the methods used which offers cautious hope for the future.

Throughout the world, but particularly in the United States and Canada, there are numerous Swallow Clubs where laryngectomy patients and their families meet monthly for practical classes and social activities.

The physiotherapist has a two-fold part to play with the laryngectomy patient. Not only will conventional treatment apply in the form of pre- and postoperative breathing exercises, neck and shoulder exercises, but also in combining with the speech therapist for controlled breathing to help prepare for the teaching of oesophageal speech and with mouth and tongue exercises to maintain mobility of movement for phonation. She can also involve herself with social rehabilitation. Even before the patient leaves hospital he should be encouraged to dress; and men should put on a collar and tie as soon as possible, so that it can be appreciated that although the tracheostomy is covered, breathing is not hindered. The first visit to a shop can be quite an ordeal and the physiotherapist may well find herself cast in the role of escort. It is not always the patient who requires such support but the well-meaning public who need the reassurance that the patient, although without his voice box, is still a human being.

Laryngectomy is seldom performed as primary treatment for cordal carcinoma, rather it is more often carried out for extensive disease involving the pharynx and/or cervical oesophagus. With this more extensive procedure there is usually a much longer recovery before speech training can even be started. It is vital that during the whole time that the patient is in hospital, he should be regularly visited by a physiotherapist so that a physically optimum condition may be maintained.

Pharyngo-laryngo-oesophagectomy with restoration of oesophageal function may take one to four months before the patient can leave the hospital. The restoration may be achieved by a colonic transplant or stomach pull-up, both these methods being done as a single stage with the excision. Another method is to reconstruct the hypopharynx and cervical oesophagus with a skin tube fashioned from the neck skin, which is achieved in two stages: total excision leaves the patient with a pharyngostome, oesophagostome and tracheostome and is followed two to three months later by the reconstruction. When this method is used, these patients require regular visits for general exercises and social reorientation. Loss of voice and lack of contact with other people can so easily cause these patients to become withdrawn. Rehabilitation must extend to the relatives, and they need to be helped to readapt themselves to changed circumstances and to understand the situation. Although patients cannot communicate vocally they will welcome listening to the homely things of life which are very much a part of normal living. They can be encouraged to play games and to use their hands, and in these matters the relatives can help. In the United States the approach to these patients is a very positive one, and from the beginning they are taught self-suctioning and self-feeding and in consequence they feel more self-reliant in a shorter time. They do not even wait for nurses to come to the bedside for dressings but take themselves to the specially designed dressing cubicles. This self-reliance is positive rehabilitation and is quite clearly the goal which should be set for every patient.

Jaw surgery

The treatment of jaw tumours inevitably results in a degree of deformity and loss of function, and it is a sad fact that many patients who have to undergo this type of surgery do not always realize the extent to which they may be affected by these deformities and mutilations. Of all types of cancer it is perhaps these affecting the mouth, tongue, mandible or maxilla that demand a team approach and consultation from the beginning, and the physiotherapist ought to be part of this team. These jaw cancers will include buccal carcinomas, tongue carcinomas, tumours of the hard palate, chondromata of mandible, sarcomata, carcinoma of tonsil and others. Many of these tumours are regarded as curable as the result of modern advances in surgical procedures; it follows that, if this is so, rehabilitation is imperative so that the patient may take up his normal life again.

Leon Gillis (1959) has written: 'those persons who are closely associated with the patient who has suffered a gross deformity from the excision of a malignant tumour must, if they are to be successful in rehabilitating him, possess a deep understanding of human nature. No-one concerned in the preparation for returning him to normal, or near normal, appearance must at any time flinch at sight of him; nor on the other hand, should the patient be regarded as a "case". It is good that he should know that many others have had a similar experience but he should also be made to feel that he is an individual and that he will be treated as an individual with sympathy for his personal problems.'

HEMI-MANDIBULECTOMY

When a simple hemi-mandibulectomy is performed, the physiotherapy is straightforward; as soon as the drains are removed, gentle encouragement in opening and closing the mouth should be practised. Provided the excision does not include the mandibular symphysis there should be no difficulties for the patient and restoration of function will be rapid. There is seldom any need to insert a prosthetic jaw replacement and resisted jaw exercises can safely be taught. The most effective way of teaching a patient to apply his own resistance is to place the back of the hand under the jaw and grade the pressure of resistance accordingly. Another method is to use a clothes peg. In both cases this should be carried out in front of a mirror so that the mouth is opened symmetrically.

When the excision includes the symphysis, a prosthesis is nearly always inserted, either at the initial operation or as a secondary procedure. When the symphysis is excised there is always a tendency to drooling from the lower lip, which makes drinking difficult and very messy. Very intensive exercises to the lips with finger assistance or resistance may be successful, but infinite patience will be required. Drinking by means of a straw will be easier than directly from a cup. Some patients learn to hold the lower lip by means of a light hold by the upper teeth or by pressure from the upper lip, and this will help to re-establish natural lip contact.

If a prosthesis is used, it is usually of a metal alloy similar to the alloys which have been developed in orthopaedic surgery (Cook, 1971).

Many cancers which involve the mandible are not confined to a circumscribed area and often involve the floor of the mouth, tongue, and possibly the cervical lymph nodes. Such an extensive operation is known as a commando procedure and can entail partial or hemi-mandibulectomy, partial glossectomy, excision of floor of mouth and block dissection of glands. Repair of the resulting defect internally is nowadays often accomplished by the use of a forehead flap and the resulting forehead deformity repaired by a graft from the thigh. A temporary tracheostomy is performed and a feeding tube passed before the patient leaves the operating theatre. When removal of involved tissue necessitates full thickness excision, then the external repair may be by means of a delto-pectoral flap with the internal lining from a forehead flap. Zirkle and Thompson (1974) describe some of these techniques.

However a reconstruction is achieved, the patient is left with marked disfigurement. They should be told not to expect rapid improvement in appearance, and as they become better adjusted, gently told that it may be all of 12 months before the new grafted skin has settled down. Plate 18 shows a female patient who underwent hemi-mandibulectomy with partial glossectomy and partial removal of the floor of mouth with a forehead flap reconstruction, and Plate 19 shows the same patient 12 months later with a changed hair-style to hide the forehead graft and a well-healed and consolidated lower jaw.

PHYSIOTHERAPY FOLLOWING JAW SURGERY

(1) Immediate postoperative chest physiotherapy.

(2) The amount of shoulder movements allowed will depend on the degree of grafting. If a forehead graft only has been used, then shoulder shrugging and circling exercises should be encouraged, which will help to relieve muscle tension. If a delto-pectoral pedicle has been raised then exercises on the affected side should be avoided, though gentle massage to the trapezius may help to ease tension. The unaffected shoulder should be exercised to maintain full movement.

(3) The patient should be encouraged to move around in bed.

(4) If radiotherapy has been given pre-operatively there may well be delayed healing, and more active massage to grafted areas and exercises for the mouth and jaw will need to be carefully graded. It is not possible to state precisely when massage or exercises may be started. It is only possible to indicate what can be done to help. A great deal of this type of rehabilitation is achieved by trial and error, and the physiotherapist should be willing to try out any of her skills. Provided the best end result is achieved, it does not matter if an unconventional method is used, provided it is discussed with the surgeon. This is why good rapport and understanding between surgeon and physiotherapist can offer so much to these patients.

MASSAGE

Forehead area. The area from which the flap is raised will be repaired by a full thickness graft probably from the thigh. When it has taken, finger kneading massage with oil or Nivea cream may be given to soften and mobilize the graft. Care must be taken at all times not to 'skin polish', but to firmly and gently knead the tissues. When the graft is firmly consolidated, gentle cupping may also be tried. The patient is treated either lying or half-lying.

External cheek grafting. Where a full thickness excision has been necessary and repaired with both a delto-pectoral graft and an internal lining, massage to the external area may commence when the stitches have been removed and the grafts have taken. The patient is treated in a lying position. The purpose of the massage is two-fold, to help disperse the oedema which is always present and to soften and mobilize the grafted area. Finger kneadings and rollings and effleurage increasing in firmness will be the techniques used.

Delto-pectoral region. The area from which the pedicle is raised may be closed by a rotation flap or by a Thiersch graft. Once healed, this area will also benefit from oil massage.

EXERCISES

Shoulders. As soon as the donor area is healed, shoulder exercises must be given to fully mobilize the shoulder joint. Free active exercises should be given with no forced movement.

Neck. Shoulder shrugging and circling exercises together with neck rotation, side flexion and circumduction may be possible from an early stage but mostly they will be limited until the grafts have taken. Again, the surgeon will indicate when they may be safely commenced.

Mouth and tongue. The patient should be encouraged to move the lips and tongue remnant as soon as possible. Oral toilet is essential for all these cases and this is a good time to suggest that the patient practise his movements. Touching the lips with ice will help to stimulate them, particularly if they are rather oedematous. Attempts at whistling and making vowel sounds all provide exercise as well as being practical.

Jaw. Once the surgeon is satisfied that the graft and jaw remnant is stable, exercises may be given to aid jaw mobility and maintain the muscles of mastication. The degree of opening of the mouth must be gently increased until it is sufficient to allow eating.

SOCIAL REHABILITATION

As soon as practical the patient should be encouraged to dress and move around the ward and hospital environs. This is the beginning of the social reorientation which can make or mar the successful operation. These patients are self-conscious and when they first venture outside the ward they should be accompanied by a nurse or physiotherapist. Indeed a visit to the physiotherapy department may be the first goal and can be used to advantage to allow the patient to join in with general classes and to have strengthening exercises such as boot and weights, springs, bicycling, etc. From the department this can be progressed to walking round the hospital and then to be taken outside into the street. The patient may have been in the ward for many months and it should be obvious that such patients cannot be discharged home without getting the feel again of people in the street, traffic generally and going on public transport, not to mention going into shops and asking for things. Speech may be permanently impaired and though speech therapy may help, patients still need to be reassured that they will be understood by the public and the only way to ensure this is to escort them discreetly. This is all part of rehabilitation and is as much the responsibility of the physiotherapist as anyone else.

Other surgical procedures which physiotherapists may encounter include maxillectomy, exenteration of the orbit, and ear surgery which can involve removal of the petrous bone. Patients who undergo excision of the hard palate will have an obturator designed for them which can be inserted immediately postoperatively. External excision of the maxilla and exenteration of the orbit require an external prosthesis, and wherever possible the cast for this should be taken before operation, or at least the patient should be seen by the prosthetic department so that he can know exactly what is being planned and provided (Thomas, 1974).

With all head and neck patients the physiotherapist must never show signs of revulsion at the sight of the mutilation. Immense patience and tact is required when treating these patients and when helping the relatives. In many cases it is the latter who require help to overcome their distaste at the situation; particularly is this true of the question of eating. After such surgery this can become a very messy affair; a liquidiser will almost certainly be required and the patient will need to experiment to find out how best to manage and what foods he can most easily manage. He should be encouraged together with his relatives to eat with them and not in seclusion (Downie, 1974).

Much of what has been written above may have sounded trite and obvious and hardly to be described as physiotherapy. However, many patients just do not receive this care and when they are discharged it becomes all too obvious that they should have received it. There is abundant evidence that physiotherapy does make a great deal of difference to the final result. The gain is not only physical but also psychological.

The following case-history describes the story of a male patient who received absolutely no physiotherapy until he reached a centre some three months after his surgery.

CASE-HISTORY

Mr. B. was a man aged 37 who had been diagnosed as having an extensive carcinoma of the lip at the right-hand side of the angle of the mouth with cervical lymph node involvement of both right and left sub-mental regions. It had been decided to treat him initially with a full course of irradiation and to follow it with radical surgery. During March and April 1971 he received this with resultant improvement to the lip area and complete resolution of the gland area.

On 31st May 1971 he was admitted for surgery and a radical resection of the right lower two-thirds of the face including a right hemi-mandibulectomy and bilateral block dissection of cervical lymph nodes was performed. The reconstruction was by a forehead flap for the lining and a delto-pectoral flap for external cover, the resultant defects being grafted as well. Mr. B. made an uneventful recovery from this; he was given a tracheostomy to ensure adequate ventilation. Between 2 June and 18 August 1971 several further operations were required to complete the major surgical procedure.

31 August 1971. Mr. B. was admitted for rehabilitation. He was noted to be a pleasant Irishman who was anxious to do everything possible to help himself. He had a tracheostomy with a silver speaking tube.

On examination. He was found to have severely restricted movements of the right shoulder. The delto-pectoral flap had been taken from the right side. There was marked oedema of the cheek graft. Direct questioning revealed:
(1) He had had absolutely no physiotherapy at any time.
(2) In 1969 he had had a 'blister' at the side of the mouth which had been biopsied and he had never been notified of the result. It later transpired that this biopsy was positive for cancer but no follow-up had been made.

Aims of treatment. Local. (1) To improve the condition of the grafted areas. (2) To improve jaw and tongue movements. (3) To restore mobility to the right shoulder.
Social. (1) To reorientate the patient back into society. (2) To ensure independence.

Plan of treatment. Local. (1) Oil massage to forehead graft. (2) Oil massage to grafted cheek area. (3) Oil massage to pectoral area. (4) Shoulder exercises, particularly pendulum swinging exercises. (5) General toning up exercises and postural correction.
Social. Daily walks with other patients and a member of staff, commencing away from the town centre and gradually progressing to areas where people would be encountered.

The grafted area in the pectoral area was paper-thin and tight and the utmost care had to be observed during massage not to 'rub' through it. The rotation of the flap extended across the shoulder and was tight, and it was for this reason that pendular exercises were considered more suitable at this stage of mobilizing the joint.

Massage to the cheek area was given largely to help reduce the oedema. The tissues were quite supple. Care was taken at all times never to drag or stretch the grafted areas.

Mr. B. was perfectly happy mixing with the other patients, but it was noticeable that when outside he would quite deliberately cross the road to avoid people. After he had been in the unit for two weeks this question of avoiding people was discussed with him at great length. At this time the unit's aide used to meet her son from school each afternoon and bring him back to the unit. Mr. B was persuaded to go with her as he already knew the boy. This proved very successful and he quickly realized that outsiders really did not stop and stare at him.

24 September 1971. Mr. B. asked if he might go to the barber for a haircut. 'I feel like a hippie' was his reason! This was a real breakthrough and from then on there was no trouble about mixing with people. By this date, shoulder mobility had increased and the pectoral grafted area was much improved and consolidated. Slings, springs and pulleys were added for the shoulder.

The oedema of the jaw had subsided and there was now good movement of the jaw.

Feeding. It was necessary for all food to be liquidised and Mr. B. was able to manage by spooning the food to the back of the mouth. Liquids such as tea, coffee, etc. he drank by using a large syringe to which he attached a wide-bore catheter and allowed the fluid to go straight down his throat.

27 September 1971. Mr. B. was admitted to the referring hospital for re-assessment and minor surgery to further correct the lip. He returned for further rehabilitation.

14 October 1971. Mr. B. developed a supraspinatus tendinitis on the right which was effectively treated with ice packs and exercises. Frictions were not possible because the skin was too thin due to the graft. The area was well oiled before applying the ice packs.

At this point the speech therapist was asked to see him in an attempt to improve his speech.

During the next two months Mr. B. underwent minor corrective surgery to the lips and face and returned between each operation to the unit. He also had the tracheostomy tube removed.

January 1972. Mr. B.'s condition was excellent. His face had settled down. He had full shoulder movement and he was waiting for the last stage of corrective surgery. Arrangements were begun to find him suitable lodgings and work prior to his ultimate discharge. The social worker at the referring hospital was extremely helpful. Mr. B. did not have a permanent home. He had been a wanderer all his life, from lodging to lodging and job to job, and clearly it was not going to be easy to find suitable living accommodation where he would also get suitable food.

February 1972. Mr. B. was finally discharged from the unit. He underwent further surgery and was discharged from hospital to a Church Army hostel.

It is pleasant to record that this patient immediately found different lodgings at a Rowton House where he was also given a job. In December 1972 he was still with them and in June 1973 he had been up-graded because his work was good.

This is a case which aptly reflects how worth while it is to ensure thorough rehabilitation in every way. It also shows plainly how long a time it takes to complete such an extensive treatment.

Chapter Nine: The role of physiotherapy in the treatment of patients undergoing surgery for miscellaneous conditions

Surgery, alone or in combination with radiotherapy or chemotherapy or both, probably remains the major treatment for a patient with oncological disease. Modern techniques of anaesthesia and postoperative care have opened up hitherto impossible pathways. Surgeons can embark on very lengthy and sophisticated operations, sure in the knowledge that the patient will be skilfully cared for afterwards. Much surgery for cancer is mutilating in the initial stages, but the patient must be reassured that reconstructive measures will be carried out to minimize its effects. This applies particularly to patients who undergo head and neck surgery and major amputations. The purpose of all surgery is to cure if possible, and, at worst, to alleviate distressing symptoms. If positive benefit from surgery is doubtful, alternative treatments will be considered.

The general principles for physiotherapy in cancer patients are the same as those for patients undergoing surgery for other diseases. These are:

(1) To prevent chest complications, by maintaining lung function and aiding the clearance of secretions.

(2) To prevent thrombosis of the legs by encouraging active leg movements, or if necessary by performing passive exercises.

(3) To maintain muscle power by encouraging simple bed exercises.

(4) To help maintain good posture by ensuring that pillows are arranged in a good supportive position.

All patients undergoing surgery should be seen pre-operatively so that a full, but simple, explanation of the proposed treatment may be given. The consultant will have explained the surgical procedures, but the physiotherapist may be able to help to clarify any problems which may arise. She will be able to offer reassurance regarding such questions as 'Will I burst my stitches when I cough?' With regard to this problem, patients should be given instruction in how to hold themselves or how to use the cough belt (Barlow, 1964).

The approach of the physiotherapist to the patient must be direct, positive and firm. Patients are very quick to sense when someone does not really know what they are doing. A sensitive yet firm hand to support an abdominal wound when coughing will not only reassure but will give confidence. The author has always found that sitting on the bed behind the patient, with the patient able to lean on her shoulder, thus enabling both her hands to be free to support the wound, is a very effective hold.

A patient who has had a thyroidectomy should be supported with one hand on the base of the occiput and the other firmly over the neck incision.

Patients who have to be given a tracheostomy should be treated in conjunction with a nurse, so that a thorough treatment may be given. It is not possible for one person to shake a patient's chest and suck out the secretions at the same time (see Plate 20).

Bladder cancer

Surgery for cancers of the bladder range from the insertion of gold grains into a small circumscribed tumour which has not invaded the muscle layer, to the radical procedure of total cystectomy with either transplant of the ureters to the rectum or the fashioning of an ileal bladder or conduit. With the latter, the ureters are transplanted into the ileum and then a loop of ileum is brought to the surface of the skin as a stoma. An appliance is permanently worn and emptied as necessary (Wallace, 1971).

When the cancer is very advanced and has invaded the uterus in a woman, or rectum in male or female, or both organs in a woman,

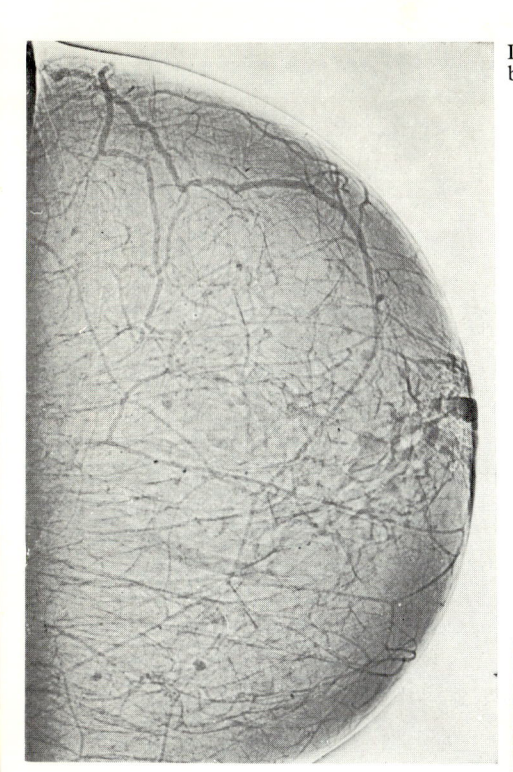

Plate 1 A xeroradiograph of a normal breast. (*See p.* 31.)

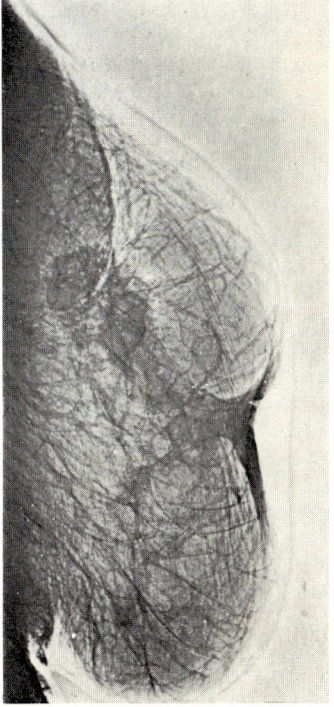

Plate 2 A xeroradiograph of a breast with an obvious tumour. Note the retracted nipple and the skin thickening. (*See p.* 31.)

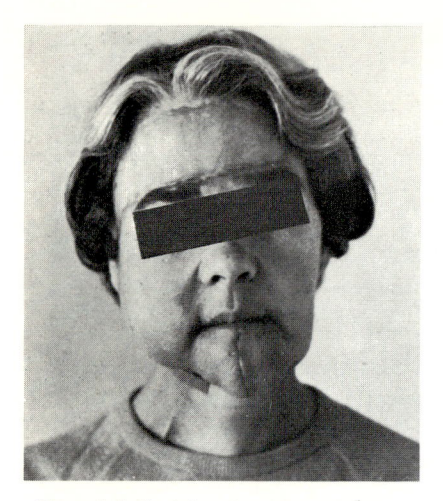

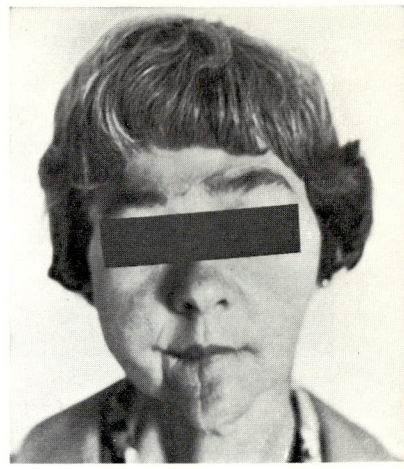

Plate 18 (*left*) A female patient who has undergone a hemi-mandibulectomy with partial glossectomy and partial removal of the floor of mouth, with repair by means of a forehead graft. Note the marked oedema of the right cheek and pronounced scarring on forehead. (*See p.* 103.)

Plate 19 (*right*) The same patient 12 months later, showing the changed hair-style to hide the forehead graft. Note also how the scarring has faded and consolidated. (*See p.* 103.)

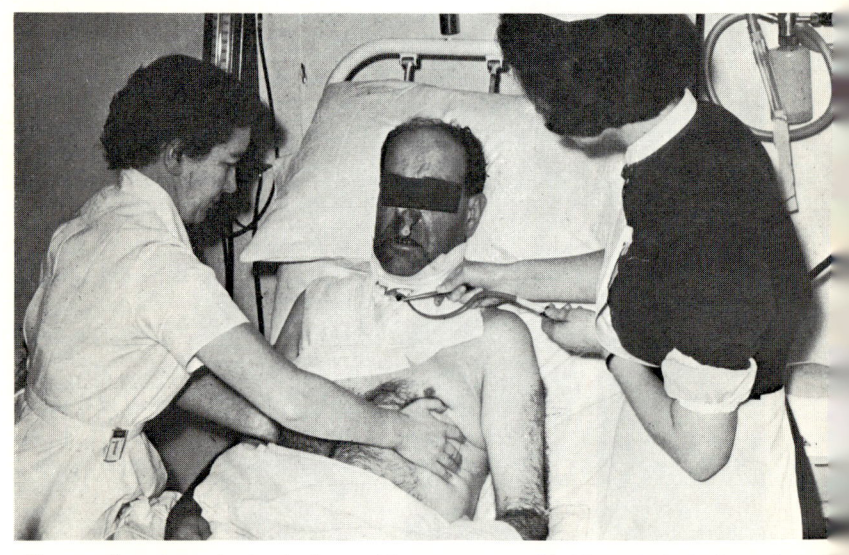

Plate 20 A patient who has had a total laryngectomy with bilateral block dissection of cervical lymph nodes, being treated by the physiotherapist whilst the nurse is giving tracheal suction. Note also the monitoring badge worn on the belt of the physiotherapist. (*See p.* 112 and 132.)

then a pelvic clearance or evisceration may be performed. Intensive investigations will first be carried out to ensure that there is no distant spread.

If the rectum is removed then the patient will of course have a colostomy in addition to the ileal conduit. In the United States an alternative has been offered in the form of a hemi-corporectomy where the body is divided at the level of lumbar 4 and 5, after an ileal conduit and colostomy have been fashioned. The added criteria would be intractable pain. The rehabilitation for such patients has been documented (Simmons, Lehman, Taylor & Delateur, 1968), and these authors have described the type of prosthesis supplied as well as the exercises and retraining required. Undoubtedly this particular form of surgery would present psychological, emotional, social as well as physical problems and physiotherapists would have an enormous part to play.

With the lesser forms of radical surgery, the general physiotherapy will be the same as for other patients undergoing major surgery, but the added experience of an artificial bladder, similar to that of colostomy following an abdominoperineal resection of rectum, does present the social problem of mixing with people again.

Whilst physiotherapists do not actually play a direct part in helping to train patients with colostomies or those with ileal conduits, indirectly they can help in a number of ways:

(1) By general exercises including abdominal exercises.

(2) By encouraging patients to dress and either walk round the hospital or its grounds, or come to the physiotherapy department and join in general classwork with other patients.

(3) By teaching them to lift; most of these patients are told not to lift heavy weights and promptly think that they cannot do anything.

(4) By showing no signs of distaste if patients show them their stomas.

(5) By showing understanding at the natural reaction of abhorrence on the part of such patients and offering reassurance in a practical way about the ability to live normally. It is useful for physiotherapists to know basic helpful hints for such patients which

they can acquire from the nursing staff, from reading, and from knowledge gained from patients themselves. As such experience grows, the physiotherapist will find herself able to offer a great deal of additional support.

There are occasions when radical cystectomy will include the excision of the symphysis pubis. These patients *will* require physical rehabilitation in the form of intensive quadriceps exercises, assisted active leg exercises including sling suspension and progressing to gait re-education. This is best started between parallel bars with subsequent progression to elbow crutches.

A firm corset will give support though care has to be taken not to compress the ileal stoma. It may be all of six to nine months before these patients can walk comfortably without sticks, and they should certainly be warned that it may take so long.

Carcinoma of the vulva

Gynaecological surgery in the main is straightforward from the point of view of treatment from the physiotherapist, but with a particular emphasis on foot and leg exercises, to prevent venous thrombosis of the legs. Occasionally, pelvic floor exercises may be necessary.

Carcinoma of the vulva, however, can require radical surgery involving excision of the vulva, lower portion of the vagina, a bilateral block dissection of the inguinal lymph nodes and in some cases a wide excision of the skin of the lower abdomen which may require skin grafting.

Apart from breathing exercises, static exercises for quadriceps and gluteal muscles should be taught, also foot exercises. Care will need to be taken so that no strain is placed on the raw areas. Quite often there is delayed healing and ultraviolet light is frequently requested.

When the patient first gets up, it will be observed that she walks with a wide base and gait re-education will be necessary together with careful postural re-education.

Vulvectomy is a most intimate operation and the feelings of

patients must be particularly respected. Depression is very common and the physiotherapist will need to be immensely understanding, patient and yet utterly firm. Diversional occupational therapy can be most helpful.

Brain and spinal surgery

Neurosurgery is usually performed in specialized units and the physiotherapist in the specialist cancer hospital, or attached to a radiotherapy unit of a general hospital, will only meet these patients if they are referred for further treatment or if they were originally patients of that hospital. This section will only give an outline of principles of treatment in the early stage since physiotherapy for such patients referred for radiotherapy has already been covered (p. 78). What must be stressed is that even if a diagnosis of a rapidly growing tumour is made, which consequently may be inoperable, or following operation may offer a very poor prognosis, the physiotherapist at that unit should still do everything to make him independent as quickly as possible and without resort to sophisticated techniques.

CRANIAL SURGERY

Primary tumours which arise in the brain affect either the nerve cells or the glial cells. Amongst the former are neuroblastomas and retinoblastomas and amongst the latter are astrocytomas, ependymomas and medulloblastomas. The aetiology of these tumours is not understood, though some may be congenital. Signs and symptoms will vary depending on the location of the tumour; following examination and the carrying out of specialized investigations such as scanning, ventriculography and angiography, the surgeon will decide whether the tumour is operable or whether irradiation is the treatment of choice.

If surgery is decided upon, a craniotomy will be performed and the extent of the tumour determined. If it is encapsulated then it may be possible to remove it entirely; often it is only possible to remove part, since to remove all would involve damaging normal brain tissue.

Following cranial surgery, the patient requires highly intensive nursing until he recovers consciousness. In the immediate postoperative period, physiotherapy will be directed towards prevention of chest complications and to the maintenance of full joint mobility of all limbs.

The degree of residual disability will depend either on how much disability was present before operation or how much damage has unavoidably occurred as the result of surgery. If there was paralysis present prior to surgery and it was possible to remove the tumour *in toto*, then there is every likelihood of complete recovery. Many of these patients will not require irradiation and their physiotherapy, if required, will follow the conventional pattern of treatments for mono- or hemiplegia. Similarly, where the tumour has been removed with some local disturbance to normal brain tissue, this may be found to be only temporary and again no permanent disability will result.

Where the tumour has not been totally removed, the patient will be referred for postoperative irradiation, and recovery of function can continue for some time even after treatment has ceased. It is interesting to note that irradiation itself sometimes leads to a worsening of a disability that is already present due to increase in oedema of the brain tissue; this is always only temporary and when it clears up the disability is found to be greatly improved.

Brain tumours are extremely variable in prognosis and if physiotherapists are required to treat a resultant disability they should be given an indication of the outcome. Some tumours can be removed and yet recur very quickly, others grow rapidly and are inoperable, whilst yet others can be removed with a good prognosis.

The utmost care must be taken when treating patients who cannot speak, and appear not to hear as the result of a brain tumour. In most cases the intellect is unimpaired and tactless remarks or discussion of his condition in his presence can be very wounding. Likewise if speech is affected, so that he speaks only with great difficulty, care must be taken not to let him feel that you regard him as dull-witted.

Rehabilitation for the brain tumour patient with a short-term prognosis must be simple and rapid to the point of maximum independence, with the family involved and knowing how much help to give. For the patient with good prognostic survival who has a disability, skilled re-education is of paramount importance. This may include a period at a rehabilitation centre and later at a re-settlement centre.

Metastases may develop in the brain, particularly from primary sites like lung, kidney or breast. Surgery may be advised for a solitary circumscribed deposit, and treatment then will be as for a primary tumour. In most cases, however, brain metastases will be treated by irradiation.

SPINAL TUMOURS

Tumours involving the spinal cord may also be primary or secondary and they may be intra- or extradural. All, in some degree, lead to compression and consequent weakness or paralysis of the limbs and trunk. Primary tumours may be ependymomas which arise from the central canal of the spinal cord and grow very slowly. Hodgkin's disease may affect the para-aortic nodes leading to extrinsic compression of the cord. Myeloma deposits may cause collapse of the vertebral bodies leading to cord compression. Secondary deposits from breast, kidney or prostate are not infrequent and they too lead to vertebral body collapse and resultant cord compression.

A myelogram may be performed to determine the level of the blockage and a decompression laminectomy carried out as soon as possible. The longer the spinal cord is compressed and the blood flow cut off, the greater will be the danger of permanent paralysis.

Practically all patients who undergo decompression laminectomy for a tumour will be given a course of postoperative irradiation and their main rehabilitation has already been discussed (see p. 67). Immediate postoperative physiotherapy however, is most important. Joint mobility must be maintained and passive movements to all paralysed limbs should be carried out at least once daily and the patient correctly positioned in bed so that deformities do not develop (Downie, 1973). Where there is active movement, it should be encouraged, and static exercises should be taught. Breathing exercises should be given and supervized at least once daily; many of these patients are in a poor state of general health and the prevention of chest complications is important.

In all cases of paralysis following spinal tumours, a wheelchair should be ordered immediately. It can be months before it is known how much recovery may occur and if none is possible, a great deal of time will have been wasted when steps could have been taken to make the patient independent in a chair. He should always be taught to understand that provision of a wheelchair is to be regarded as a precautionary measure.

Neurosurgical physiotherapy is therefore most important for these patients in the immediate postoperative period, prior to the transfer for irradiation. It should always have the two-fold objects of prevention of chest complications and the prevention of contractures by ensuring joint mobility.

CASE-HISTORY

Mrs. O. was an accountant aged 61 who had originally been treated in 1955 for breast cancer. She had undergone mastectomy followed by irradiation and had made an uneventful recovery. In April 1972 her back suddenly 'gave way' and five days later she noticed weakness of her legs. In May she twice collapsed to the floor and was finally admitted to a neurosurgical unit for assessment and a decompression laminectomy. Operation revealed a tumour in the region of dorsal 5 which, on histological examination and comparison with the primary tumour histology, showed it to be a secondary deposit from the breast tumour of 17 years previously. Mrs. O. was referred for radiotherapy and afterwards was admitted to a rehabilitation centre for intensive treatment, particularly with a view to going home.

23 June 1972. On admission a review of Mrs. O.'s past history revealed several facts which were particularly relevant to the physiotherapist.

(1) As an adolescent she had sustained severe scalds to her right hand which had necessitated amputation of the index finger. The hand was severely deformed and the skin in a poor condition.

(2) In 1965 she had undergone laminectomy for a lumbar disc lesion and was left with residual weakness of the right leg with complete foot drop.

(3) In 1970 systemic lupus erythematosus was diagnosed and this exacerbated the skin condition of the right hand. (Systemic lupus erythematosus is sometimes a manifestation of latent malignant disease.)

On examination it was apparent that Mrs. O. was a courageous, sensible and intelligent patient who was quite determined to become independent and return home. She also let it be clearly known that she understood her disease and the future, and was obviously well-adjusted mentally.

Physical examination. There was a full range of movement in all joints of the upper and lower limbs with the exception of the right ankle joint which had been useless since the 1965 laminectomy. There was good and equal power in the upper limbs. Table 1 shows a comparison of the muscle power in both limbs, on admission and on discharge. It will be noted that in all affected groups there is improvement.

Mrs. O. was mobile in bed in that she was able to sit up from the lying position and roll from side to side. She had previously been allowed to walk *badly* with one stick and the support of one person. It was explained to Mrs. O. that the aims of treatment would be (1) to strengthen leg muscles; (2) to improve balance; (3) to re-educate walking and progress to stairs; (4) to make her independent within her own limitations.

The present method of walking was stopped by the consultant, who explained to Mrs. O. that she would be re-educated in walking in the parallel bars and, when her balance improved, then and then only would walking be permitted outside the physiotherapy department. It was also agreed that initially Mrs. O. would have four weeks of rehabilitation and that immediate steps would be taken get her rehoused into a ground-floor flat. There was excellent liaison with the referring hospital and they undertook all the necessary social work.

Table I Comparison of muscle power on admission and on discharge

	Right		Left	
	26 June 1972	2 August 1972	26 June 1972	2 August 1972
Hips				
Flexion	3+	4	4	4+
Extension	4+	5	5	5
Abduction	3	3+	3+	4
Adduction	3	3+	3+	4
Int. rotation	3+	4	4	4
Ext. rotation	2+	3	3+	3+
Knees				
Flexion	2	2+	3	3+
Extension	3+	4+	4	5
Ankles				
Plantarflexion	2+	3+	5	5
Dorsiflexion	0	0	5	5
Inversion	0	0	5	5
Eversion	0	0	5	5
Balance				
Sitting	Fair	Good		
Standing	Poor	Fair		

First week. (1) General classwork, sitting in wheelchair with special emphasis on general mobility.

(2) Transfers taught from bed to chair, and back, using a transfer board. By the end of the week the patient could do this easily without external assistance. (This was the goal set for the first week).

(3) General leg exercises. Static quadriceps exercises over a pillow and knee flexion and extension actively over the side of the bed.

(4) Rhythmic stabilizations in the sitting positions to improve balance.

(5) Gait training between the parallel bars.

The accent was on active exercises because the patient expressed the desire to be able to practise during the evening. Proprioceptive neuromuscular facilitation techniques were used but were kept to a minimum.

Second week. (1) Classwork continued, but was now regarded as 'limbering up' as well as an occasion for good-natured bullying with the other patients. The arms were removed from the wheelchair.

(2) Arm exercises using spring resistance to strengthen upper arms and shoulder girdle so that progression could be made in transferring from bed to chair, and chair to lavatory, without the use of the transfer board. (This was the goal for the second week.)

(3) Active quadriceps exercises over a wedged pillow.

(4) Rhythmic stabilizations in standing between the parallel bars as well as in sitting.

(5) Walking with elbow crutches was begun; the right-hand grip was well padded so that an adequate hold was achieved.

Third week. (1) Classwork, but the patient was now able to sit on an ordinary chair.

(2) Leg exercises continued but with some manual resistance increasing to light springs by the end of the week.

(3) The ordinary elbow crutches were exchanged for forearm support crutches (gutter crutches) which were found to be much more comfortable and manageable. The skin over the knuckles of the right hand had already begun to give cause for concern and changing to gutter crutches removed the strain of gripping.

(4) Balance control was now much improved and Mrs. O. found she could put on her pants, trousers, shoes and socks with no difficulty. (This was the goal for the third week.)

(5) In the first and second weeks Mrs. O. had managed to do the washing up and drying whilst in the wheelchair. She now found that she could stand for the washing up.

Fourth week. (1) Mrs. O. was now able to walk slowly and confidently up to a hundred yards. She was now taught to negotiate stairs using one crutch and the banister. Mrs. O. was going to a friend's home before returning to her own and it was necessary that she should be able to manage some stairs.

(2) Progression to straight leg raising with boot and one-pound weight (10 × 3) and over the side of the bed with two-pound weight (10 × 3).

(3) During this week a home visit was made to the house where Mrs. O. was going. The ground floor and the first floor presented no problems. The bathroom and lavatory were satisfactory, but the stairs were steep and awkward. Prudence won the day and, rather than pointing out the ghastly difficulties, a suggestion that two additional hand grips be fixed was gladly and gratefully accepted. It was agreed that Mrs. O. should try a weekend at the house and if all was satisfactory then she would be discharged.

This plan was duly carried out and on 12 August 1972 Mrs. O. was discharged. Arrangements were made for domiciliary physiotherapy twice weekly and, in addition, simple equipment was lent to Mrs. O. so that she might continue to carry out her exercises daily.

September 1972. Mrs. O. returned to her own home.

Bone surgery and amputations

Tumours of bone are not common, but alas, are always very serious and mostly require radical amputation if there is to be any hope of even limited success in controlling the disease. Osteosarcoma, osteochondroma, fibrosarcoma, Ewing's tumour (giant cell tumour) are but a few of the types of tumour which may be encountered and they mostly affect the long bones. They occur most frequently in children and young adults who invariably complain of swelling and pain which does not go with the rest. These primary bone tumours are usually rapid in growth and metastasise to the lungs. The primary treatment is usually irradiation followed by amputation six months later. The reason for the delay is that it is possible by then to see whether there are signs of pulmonary deposits, and the pre-operative irradiation also reduces the risk of tumour cells being spread in the bloodstream.

If there is no evidence of lung deposits, amputation will be performed. If the tumour is anywhere in the femur a hip disarticulation or hindquarter amputation will be necessary. If the tibia is affected, an above-knee amputation will be performed. If there is a tumour in the humerus, a shoulder disarticulation or forequarter amputation will be carried out.

Amputation may also be required in soft tissue tumours, e.g. chronic squamous cell carcinoma which ulcerates, or malignant melanoma.

THE ROLE OF THE PHYSIOTHERAPIST

There is no doubt that the physiotherapist should be involved with any potential amputation patient in the pre-operative period. Once amputation is decided upon, the patient requires all the support and help possible. He should be seen pre-operatively at the limb fitting centre and should see exactly what type of prosthesis he will have. It is possible sometimes to take measurements pre-operatively so that the prosthesis can be ready postoperatively as soon as the surgeon decides the patient is fit to start wearing the prosthesis. Pre-operatively the physiotherapist should teach the patient how to handle a pair of crutches for walking and stair climbing. This will save much time afterwards and enables the patient to appreciate that 'something' is being done.

POSTOPERATIVE CARE

Following amputation of a lower limb for malignancy, the physiotherapy will be exactly the same as for amputation for other causes and it is not intended to describe this.

Disarticulation of the hip and hemi-pelvectomy will not require bandaging, but these patients will require greater help in regaining balance control. Once the drains are removed ambulation can proceed and walking is best commenced between bars before progressing to elbow crutches. As most of these patients are young there is seldom any difficulty in mobilizing them. By the end of three weeks they should be ready to go to the limb fitting centre for measurement, if not already done, or for a preliminary fitting. Whilst waiting for the limb to be made, a concentrated programme of more strenuous exercises can be taught if the general health of the patient allows. Extended distance walking will help to keep the normal leg in good tone. The patient should be encouraged from the beginning to continue to live as actively and normally as possible. When the limb is ready for the final fitting the patient will usually be taught to walk with it at the limb fitting centre. As well as learning to walk and climb stairs, it is as well to find out if there is anything particular that the patient wishes to be able to do. An active churchgoer will require to kneel and genuflect; a tourist guide may need to be able to walk over cobbles and rough land; a surveyor may need to get up and down narrow stairs, etc. It is these extra things which will count in the final estimate of whether a patient is fully rehabilitated.

Above- and below-knee amputations will require careful bandaging and adequate care to prevent contracture. Where irradiation has been given, delayed healing may be encountered and this may delay either fitting or measuring of the limb. Adequate bandaging cannot really commence until healing has taken place. As soon as possible these patients should be mobilized on elbow crutches.

Prognosis may be comparatively short for some of these patients, and the accent must be on rapid activation. It is greatly to be hoped that at least a pylon will be available from the very earliest moment postoperatively. In some cases the making of a definitive limb may not be justified, but the provision of a pylon for above- and below-knee amputations is essential.

As with other amputees, the patient will require much support and understanding. The loss of a limb is not only physically traumatic, it is emotionally traumatic and patients do feel justifiably angry at the loss of part of their body. With young adults, and more particularly with children, the relatives will need much help to adjust. They must be helped not to be over-protective, but to understand how important it is to allow the patient to become independent, e.g. if he falls they must not rush to pick him up but help him to do it himself.

SECONDARY DEPOSITS IN BONE

As well as primary tumours, secondary deposits from breast, kidney, prostate, pancreas, thyroid and other sites can appear in any bone in the body. Deposits in the weight-bearing bones can lead to pathological fractures, and indeed it is not uncommon for a patient to be admitted with a fracture which is found to be pathological and is the first indication of a cancer somewhere else. Most of these pathological fractures are treated with intramedullary nailing, or sometimes, in the case of a fracture in the neck of femur, by a prosthetic replacement such as an Austin Moore or Thompson prosthesis. The metastatic deposit is also usually irradiated and this may delay weight-bearing.

Thoracic surgery

Cancers involving the bronchi are extremely common and they occur mostly in male patients, although the incidence in females is rising rapidly. Unfortunately many of these patients are diagnosed at a late stage and are only able to receive palliative treatment, usually in the form of irradiation.

Physiotherapists may well be asked to treat such patients and particularly to teach them controlled breathing and to help them cough up secretions. Many of them will be ill and debilitated and will not be able to tolerate long tiring treatments. 'Little and often' should be the approach to treatment for such patients. The use of intermittent positive pressure breathing (IPPB) may be advised, but this must only be used on the direct referral of a doctor. Friar's balsam inhalations immediately prior to treatment can be helpful.

Thoracic surgery is almost always carried out in specific thoracic units, and only the bare outlines of aims and methods are given here.

Thoracotomy will be the first stage to allow the surgeon to assess the extent of disease. If he finds that it is too advanced for removal, the incision will be closed in layers and the patient referred for either palliative irradiation or possibly chemotherapy.

If surgery is feasible, and depending upon the extent of the disease, either a lobectomy or pneumonectomy will be performed.

Prior to any thoracic surgery, lung function tests will have been carried out to assess the lung capacity and much will depend upon these findings as to how extensive the surgery will be. Sometimes the pericardium may be invaded and this will require localized stripping; sometimes a local area of the rib cage may be affected and parts of the ribs will need to be excised also.

PRINCIPLES OF PHYSIOTHERAPY TREATMENT

These are well-known to all physiotherapists and are summarized as follows:

(1) To maintain adequate ventilation.

(2) To aid removal of secretions and thereby help to prevent pulmonary collapse.

(3) To maintain full expansion of the remaining lung in the case of pneumonectomy, and to help regain full expansion of the affected lung in the case of lobectomy.

(4) To prevent thrombosis of the legs.

(5) To prevent postural deformity.

(6) To restore exercise tolerance and help the patient regain independence.

(7) To help the relatives understand the limitations of the patient's ability, when necessary.

PRE-OPERATIVE TREATMENT

As in all pre-operative care, a simple straightforward explanation of what will be required of the patient is the first priority. He should be strongly reassured that neither breathing, coughing nor moving will in any way damage his stitches. He should be warned that inevitably these actions will cause some pain, but that adequate analgesics will be given. He should also be shown how he may hold himself when coughing, and it must be impressed upon him

PHYSIOTHERAPY IN MISCELLANEOUS CONDITIONS

how very important it is that he practises his breathing and coughs up any sputum.

Breathing exercises which need to be taught are (1) diaphragmatic breathing and (2) bilateral and unilateral basal breathing with particular emphasis on the incision side, unless it is known for certain that a pneumonectomy is to be performed.

The range of shoulder movements needs to be assessed and noted and simple exercises taught.

Foot and leg exercises should be taught and the patient encouraged to carry them out hourly during the waking hours.

POSTOPERATIVE TREATMENT

In a straightforward resection, either lobectomy or pneumonectomy, the postoperative care is routine. The patient may be treated in side-lying and Fig. 1 shows a suitable supportive hold to encourage coughing, thus combining physiotherapy with nursing procedures. Vibrations and shakings are more suitable than clapping. If a pneumonectomy has been carried out, the patient

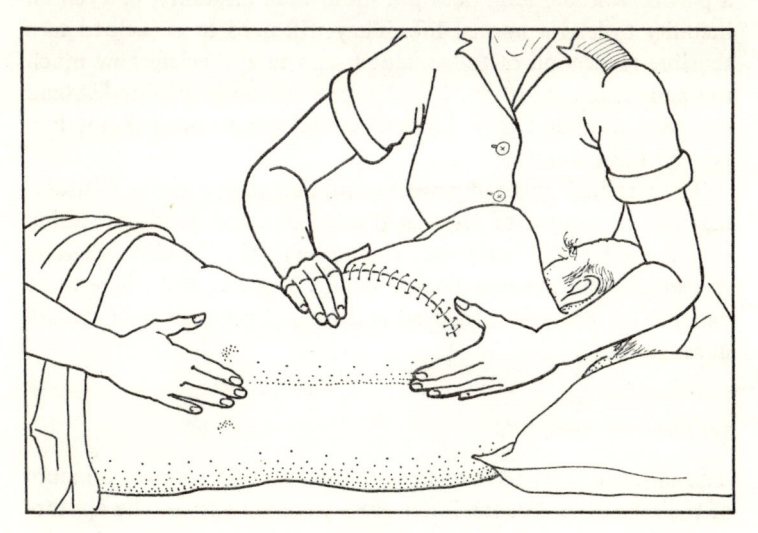

Fig. 1

may be treated lying on his incisional side, and if he has an intercostal drain, this must be securely clamped before he coughs; in fact, the drain will probably be clamped all the time and only released for short periods at specified intervals. If the clamping of the tube is not observed, a very marked mediastinal shift can occur, causing the patient severe pain and requiring the instillation of air to stabilize the pressures.

When rib resections have also been necessary, modified treatment may be needed and the patient may have a tracheostomy. The physiotherapist should be guided by the doctor as well as by her own observations.

All thoracic patients should be mobilized as soon as possible and graded walking encouraged. Sometimes a pattern of breathing whilst walking or climbing stairs will help. Many patients operated on for lung cancer have a short prognosis and the aim must be maximum exercise tolerance and independence as quickly as possible. The physiotherapist's encouragement, enthusiasm and reassurance will do much to help.

Many relatives and friends need to understand that resection of a part or a whole lung does not mean total disability, or even an inability to lead a normal life. They will need to be helped to a sensible realization of the situation, and to appreciate how much the patient is able to do. Equally, patients must also understand the need to accept their limitations and not to push themselves beyond these limits.

The terminal stages of patients with lung cancer can be distressing, and it remains to say that if relaxation and gentle breathing exercises offer help, then they should be given. No physiotherapy treatment that increases distress should be given, and where these patients are comatose, tracheal suction and postural drainage are never justified.

SECONDARY DEPOSITS

The above remarks have referred to treatment for primary tumours of the bronchus, but the lungs are a common site for the appearance of secondary deposits, just as they themselves often give rise to secondary deposits, often in the brain. With a single deposit in the lung that can be determined by whole lung tomography, and a patient who is obviously fit and with no evidence of any disease elsewhere, resection of the deposit may be carried out. The physiotherapy treatment will be exactly the same as that described above.

Chapter Ten: **Precautions to be understood, undertaken or observed by physiotherapists when treating patients for cancer**

Many people are still under the misapprehension that patients with a cancerous disease are infectious or contagious; this is not true and physiotherapists need have no fear of treating these patients. Indeed, it is important not to look upon them as being something different from others.

SHORT-WAVE DIATHERMY

Some textbooks state that patients suffering from cancer should not be given short-wave diathermy. Until more research is carried out, it is probably wiser not to give it directly to the tumour area. If, however, the particular patient is suffering from both breast cancer *and* a proven osteo-arthritic knee for which short-wave diathermy is prescribed, the latter treatment can be safely carried out. In other words, common sense and consultation between surgeon or physician and physiotherapist should enable these individual problems to be resolved.

BACK PAIN

Patients referred to physiotherapy departments with 'back ache' which does not respond to treatment, should be treated with care. A number of cancer patients present with backache, which on examination does not fit into a well-defined pattern of symptoms. It is true to say that the patient may complain of pain and yet on examination be found to have a full, free and painless range of movements. Early secondary bone deposits seldom show on X-ray examination. One case-history is recalled as typical.

Mr. X. was a patient who had advanced bladder cancer but his immediate past history was salutary. He had been referred initially to a physiotherapy department where a prolapsed intervertebral lumbar disc had been diagnosed. He was treated with traction, manipulation and short-wave diathermy with no improvement. Whilst undergoing treatment he had developed bladder symptoms and was referred to a urologist where cystoscopy showed an advanced bladder cancer and a lumbar spine X-ray (his first) showed collapse of the third and fourth vertebrae. He was immediately admitted to a specialist hospital where surgery was undertaken for the bladder cancer and radiotherapy given for the lumbar spine deposits. He made a good recovery and was able to return, pain-free, to work, albeit for only a short time.

This is *not* an isolated case, and it cannot be overstressed that if physiotherapists are asked to treat patients with back pain anywhere from the cervical region to the sacrum, and are not happy with the symptoms or with the progress, they *must* go to the consultant concerned and express their concern. Cyriax (1971) describes simply and clearly examination techniques which can form guidelines for all physiotherapists.

Radiotherapy precautions

Stringent precautions for everyone working directly or indirectly with radioactive materials are laid down in the *Radioactive Substances Act, 1948*. One of these precautions is the wearing of monitoring badges, which record on an X-ray film the amount of radiation to which a person may have been exposed. If a physiotherapist is required to wear one, she will first fill in a form relating to personal details and undergo a medical examination which will include a blood test. This information is ultimately filed in a central record office. The badge is changed regularly, developed, and the amount of recorded radiation is charted on the personal file. In this way an accurate record is maintained for all personnel working with or near radioactive material. Not every hospital where radioactive materials are in use insist that the physiotherapist wears a badge. A physiotherapist has the right, however, if she is unhappy, to consult with the Radiological Protection Adviser as to the desirability of wearing a badge. Pregnant staff certainly should not be expected to work with or near patients who are radioactive. Because of the method of central filing it is possible for people to be carefully monitored from hospital to hospital. The badge should be worn on the belt of the overall or pocket. (Plate 20 shows a physiotherapist wearing such a badge on the overall belt.)

Note. Whilst on the subject of radiation, it may be apt to comment on the problem experienced by some physiotherapists in intensive care units. Frequently, chest X-rays are required on these patients and physiotherapists become involved in holding the plate behind the patient; likewise they may be treating a patient in the next bed to a patient being X-rayed. Both these situations are to be deplored. Physiotherapists should not hold X-ray plates and they should move from the bedside while X-rays are being taken.

INTERNAL IRRADIATION PRECAUTIONS

Intra-cavitary irradiation. Carcinoma of the cervix is generally treated with intra-cavitary radium or caesium. If physiotherapy is required, the time which can safely be spent with the patient will be clearly indicated on the radiation board at the foot of the bed. This *must* be observed. The boards are yellow in colour with the radiation symbol on them.

Physiotherapy is seldom required for these patients, but if it is, it should be requested directly by the consultant or senior registrar. Intra-cavitary radium of caesium is generally only in situ for 18 to 20 hours and as soon as it is removed there is absolutely no danger of irradiation. Whilst the intra-cavitary insertions are in situ, physiotherapists should remember not to linger at the bedside of patients on either side of the treated patient.

Radioactive grains. Radioactive grains are usually of gold and are used as the treatment for small circumscribed tumours of the bladder, as palliative treatment for carcinomas of the head of pancreas which are inoperable, and as one of the treatments available for small tumours of the head and neck.

Gold grains have a short half-life and, again, the yellow board at the foot of the bed will indicate the maximum time which may be spent at the bedside. This time will increase each day over a period of four to five days, by which time the radioactivity will be negligible.

Provided these times are observed there is *no* danger to physiotherapists who may well have to treat these patients.

Radioactive needles. Radioactive needles are usually of radium or caesium and are mainly used for treating tongue and cheek cancers. Because they are relatively superficially placed physiotherapists must *never* treat these patients except on a direct and very special request from the consultant. One of the additional dangers with needles is that they may become loose and be coughed out.

They will be in situ for seven to ten days, but once removed there is again no danger and any physiotherapy can safely be undertaken. During the period when the needles are in situ, the patient is not allowed to walk about.

Liquid radioactive material. Radioactive gold in liquid form may be instilled into the pleura or peritoneum for the control of malignant fluid. In order that this may be most effective, postural drainage and positioning will be necessary and the physiotherapist may well be asked to help, particularly with the chest patients. To achieve the correct dosage the amount of time that the patient needs to spend in any one position will have been carefully worked out by the physicist and listed. Provided that the rules stated above are observed, there is no danger to the physiotherapist.

Whenever internal irradiation is used as a treatment, and the patient requires physiotherapy, there need be no fear on the part of the physiotherapist *provided* she observes the safety rules. In all hospitals where there is a great use of radioactive treatments, there will be a Radiological Protection Adviser and if there are any doubts the physiotherapist should seek his advice.

EXTERNAL IRRADIATION

There are no direct precautions to be observed by the physiotherapist in the treating of patients receiving external irradiation. Such treatment may, however, be a contra-indication to the use of some physiotherapeutic treatments.

Short-wave diathermy, microwave, infra-red, radiant heat or ultraviolet light must not be used on the area directly under external irradiation treatment. This restriction should be observed for at least three months after treatment ceases so that the local reaction is allowed to subside. It is possible to carry out ultraviolet light (UVL) treatment to an indolent area or a pressure sore within the limits of the field of radiation, provided that the raw area has been shielded from the radiation and the UVL treatment is strictly localized.

After some months, if patients who have undergone external irradiation are referred for physiotherapeutic treatments such as short-wave diathermy, or other forms of heat treatment, to the area previously irradiated, very careful skin testing must be carried out. Frequently there is marked alteration in sensation and this must be carefully checked.

No patient should undergo hydrotherapy treatments either during the external irradiation treatment or for some weeks afterwards, until the skin reaction has subsided and the consultant gives the 'all clear' for such treatment.

The reason for these precautions is quite simply that external irradiation may have a direct effect upon the peripheral circulation, leading to a diminished response to the local body-heat regulation mechanism. The skin may also become extremely sore and any additional heat will lead to increased irritation and discomfort.

If a physiotherapist is instructed to treat such a patient despite pointing out the possible dangers, she must be absolutely certain that no blame will be attached to her if the treatment leads to a worsening of the situation. In such cases, the absolute minimum dose should be given. It may well be argued that physiotherapists will have a Consultant in Physical Medicine who will be responsible for the prescribing of such treatments, but this is not so in some specialized units in the United Kingdom, nor in units abroad.

Chemotherapy

Some chemotherapeutic drugs can lead to increased photosensitivity and if a patient is referred for general UVL treatment this fact must be remembered. If the prescribing physician is unable to tell the physiotherapist whether the particular drug or drugs is a sensitizer, the pharmacist should be consulted and if there is any doubt he will be able to contact the manufacturer. Do *not* be tempted to take a risk, for the reaction can be devastating. This applies also to natural sunlight, and a case is vividly recalled where an outpatient receiving chemotherapy went to the seaside for a day trip with her husband and ended up in the local hospital with acute sunburn.

Surgery

If a patient with bone secondaries in the ribs, sternum or dorsal spine undergoes surgery, care will need to be observed when postoperative chest physiotherapy is carried out. Gentle vibrations and rollings will be preferable to heavy shakings and clapping. Postural drainage should be within the limits of the patient's tolerance and quite often the change from sitting to lying is enough.

Many cancer patients who undergo surgery are in a poor general state and all physiotherapy treatments will need to be adapted to the patient's condition. Firmness tempered with compassion should be the keynote to the physiotherapist's approach and when possible the main treatments should be combined with the nursing procedures.

Chapter Eleven: The place of physiotherapy in the care of the terminally ill and those with pain problems

It is often said that once a patient has reached the end of active treatment from the medical standpoint then there is nothing else that a physiotherapist can offer. This is not true, for if patients have been known and treated over a number of years, or even for only a short time, it is most unkind to forget them at the time when they require all the help that can be offered. Complicated treatments are certainly not advocated but with perception and adroitness it *is* possible to help many patients to the point of death.

Nowadays, death is almost a taboo subject. Why this is so is inexplicable, for by its very nature death is a most natural thing; coupled with life it remains the twin absolute certainty which applies to every person. Guardini (1954) writes that death is not merely an appendix to life in the manner of the ending of a bad play that might turn out anyhow. Death is built into life's structure and issues from its course. It is present long before the conclusion, actually throughout the whole development of life. Life has been defined as a moment directed towards death. The physiotherapist who works with cancer patients must accept that a number of patients are going to die and that she will be involved and in some cases will indeed be the one who offers the greatest support to a particular patient, though she may never know this.

In the care of the dying patient common sense and experience will govern the majority of decisions, and a sure faith and understanding of people will help. If a patient has been in the care of an understanding team whom he trusts, this latter stage will fall more naturally into place. It is when there is a sudden deterioration and the patient and relatives are unprepared, that difficulties can arise. It is well to remember that these patients, while not minding being alone, do fear loneliness almost more than anything else. Often they require only someone to sit with them and to listen to their expressions of feelings and thoughts. Who they choose to do this with is their own concern, but it may well be the physiotherapist, and time-consuming though it is, it is a task which must be fulfilled willingly.

'Am I dying?' At first sight, how difficult to answer, but experience shows that seldom is it asked in such a direct manner and seldom does the patient require an answer; rather does he or she wish to go further and express all sorts of other matters. Confidences uttered at these times must be strictly maintained, although if it is felt that more adequate help could be forthcoming from another source, the patient's permission should be sought.

As death approaches, patients are less and less able to make adjustments, and this again is why they look for the familiar face. Gradual acceptance of the ultimate will come but each person must meet this in his own way and no one of us can really imagine how someone else will react. Certainly, as death approaches we must be aware of the temptation to impose our own ideas on them. 'The only suffering of which we can fully or ultimately be aware is our own. It is true that by imaginative sympathy we can, to some extent, understand what other people are feeling... All we are generally capable of understanding is an experience of our own, in the past. We feel or live their sufferings by refeeling or reliving our own. If somebody suffers in a way in which we have never suffered, we may indeed know that they are suffering, but we shall be unable to feel with them because what they are feeling is to us a closed book' (Williams, 1972).

Physiotherapy for the truly dying patient must be limited therefore to something which the patient can comprehend and wishes to do. In such cases the physiotherapist will probably have to do the greater portion of the work and yet the help given must be unobtrusive. A calm, confident and realistic approach to life sums up the approach which a physiotherapist should show to the dying patient.

There is another side to this difficult question and one which can lead to much heartsearching. What does the physiotherapist do when asked to treat a dying patient for the first time? In particular, one thinks of the patient who has widespread disseminated disease, who develops pneumonia and a request for chest physiotherapy is made. The first criterion should be, by treating the patient will he die more peacefully? If this is so, then treat him. The second criterion is the more personal assessment of whether you would allow your own parents to be treated in such a situation. If the answer is again yes, then one should treat the patient. Many treatments are given to the terminally ill for the express purpose of enabling them to die more peacefully, and physiotherapy may, on occasion, come into this category. If, however, a physiotherapist is unhappy about such treatments then she must say so. If she has been accepted as part of a team, then this is one of the problems which requires a team discussion and a joint solution.

Then there is the comment so often expressed by physiotherapists, 'I have to treat a terminal patient every day and I could use the time more profitably on other patients'. It is not for any one of us to say that a patient will not recover; quite unaccountable things do happen and it is necessary and right that physiotherapists should accept and play their part in this aspect of patient care as fully as possible.

If one is priviliged to partake in the work of any of the specialist hospices for the dying, it becomes patently clear that the goal for each patient is simply to live each day as it comes, and for the physiotherapist this will certainly mean adjusting her treatments for individual patients on a daily basis. Sister Magdalen (1974) has written, 'very sick people are sent to us from hospitals and home towards the end of what is often a long drawn-out illness. There has been, in general, that emphasis on physical recovery which obscures the truth. It remains for us to win their confidence, to give them a security which comes from the sense of belonging to a family, so that we can live each day as a little life which is shared as we move through it together. It is part of a logical sequence in which we may find all our potentialities, come what may. It is for us to listen and learn to understand the unspoken word and the least indication of need'.

All physiotherapists would do well to ponder those words and decide where their skills could be utilized. Certainly massage can give great physical relief to aching limbs and allows that time 'to listen' as well as 'learning to understand the unspoken word'.

EUTHANASIA

Even today, many people equate dying of cancer with dying in agony, and from time to time the question of euthanasia is raised. It is as well for physiotherapists to be aware of this, to understand the implications, and to be prepared to speak out fearlessly against it. Nowadays pain control, both physical and mental, is better understood; pain is more able to be treated adequately and should not therefore present problems. The positive answer to euthanasia is education of this aspect, and reassurance to the public that such treatment is possible.

The word euthanasia is derived from a Greek word meaning 'peaceful death', but the modern connotation implies the deliberate ending of a person's life. In 1973 Cardinal Heenan stated the Christian teaching on the care of the incurably ill as follows:

> It is not for me to give medical and legal arguments against euthanasia. Nor shall I discuss the social implications of killing sick people whether with or without their consent. I do not intend to deal with those for whom men are high-grade animals without responsibility to any law not made by man. It is my task to give briefly the Christian teaching on treatment of the incurably sick.
>
> (1) The first principle is that Almighty God as the author of life is also the Lord of life. God alone is Creator. Parents are called pro-creators. That is our way of saying that they are not absolute in their authority over the life they bring in the world. This is a fundamental truth accepted by all civilized societies until our own day.

(2) The second principle is that no private person has the right to destroy life whether his own or another's.

(3) Thirdly, there are legitimate differences of opinion among believers regarding the rights of the State over life. In general terms these concern killing in war and in peace. Not all agree that the State can authorize the killing (a) of aggressors by force of arms and (b) of criminals by execution. Some Christians hold that killing is legitimate in a just war or in self-defence. Pacificists regard no price as too high to pay for peace. They deny the right and duty of the State to maintain military defences. Some Christians, who are not necessarily pacificists, hold that the capital punishment of criminals is immoral.

(4) Direct killing of the incurably sick, disabled or insane is never justified.

(5) The Catholic Church condemns the direct killing of the living foetus although saving the life of the mother may indirectly involve the death of the foetus.

(6) It is not permissible to withold nourishment or normal medical aids with the object of hastening a patient's death.

It is not for the theologian to define in detail what is meant by normal medical aids. The kiss-of-life or mechanical resuscitation of a patient suffering from shock would now be regarded as normal. The prolonged use of machines to maintain the action of heart or lungs though commonplace would be regarded as extra-ordinary means of preserving life. In certain circumstances such means might and perhaps ought to be discontinued on ethical grounds.

The patient and the doctor have different responsibilities. It may be the duty of doctor and relatives to provide the opportunity of treatment to save or prolong life. It may be their duty in the old phrase 'to allow nature to take its course'. It is not the duty of the patient to accept treatment which will purchase a further lease of life at the cost of great suffering or discomfort. Thus it would be unethical for the surgeon merely for the sake of research to persuade a patient to submit to an operation which might save the patient from death only to survive in misery.

For the Christian there are many fates worse than death. Often death is the last friend rather than the last enemy. In the *Canterbury Tales* Chaucer says, 'Death is an end of every worldly sore.' Shelley also pays tribute to death: 'How wonderful is Death, Death and his brother sleep!' Death is not a misfortune to be warded off at all costs. The death of God's friends is precious in His sight because it is a homecoming. That is why we need not hesitate to alleviate pain merely from fear of bringing nearer the hour of death. It is good ethics to ensure the comfort of the dying. It disposes of the chief argument in support of euthanasia.

The moral sense and compassion of doctors and nurses must decide what is for the patient's good. It is not euthanasia to refuse to use extra-ordinary methods to conquer a critical condition in a patient already suffering from a chronic terminal illness. To help patients to die in peace and dignity is part of the art of nursing and medicine.

These are the general principles. If we depart from them either to co-operate in suicide or to execute incurables we trespass on God's province and run the risk of destroying the whole moral law. With the decline of religion people have already begun to confuse legality with morality. Abortion and homosexual practices are regarded by many as morally acceptable because they are now permitted by law. If euthanasia were to become legal no sick or old person would be safe. The law of God is also the law of reason.

These are clear facts which should help all physiotherapists to better understand the very real difficulties which can arise in caring for the dying. It is an issue which cannot be evaded and one with which all right-thinking professionals should be concerned. It is probably true to say that it is not death itself which people fear, it is the process of dying and the very real fear of being subjected to unpleasant treatments with no real purpose save that of satisfying medical science. If this latter fear can be confidently resolved, and the patient and his family convinced and reassured that he will neither be allowed to suffer pain nor be regarded as useless and a nuisance, then the question of euthanasia should not even be contemplated.

True care for the dying patient does not involve sophisticated medical treatments; it demands care, understanding and compassion of the very highest standards, and for all of us in the caring professions it must ever remain the supreme test. For the physiotherapist it must never be regarded as a waste of time.

CASE-HISTORY

Mrs. M. was a lady of 53 who in 1967 had had a left radical mastectomy followed by irradiation. The pathology report described an adenocarcinoma with axillary gland involvement. Between February 1968 and July 1971 she received various courses of irradiation for secondary bone deposits in the spine, pelvis and ribs. An oophorectomy was performed but she declined an adrenalectomy. She was given Durabolin and cortisone. In August 1971 she developed pneumonia and was subsequently diagnosed as having secondary deposits in the lungs. Following a family discussion it was agreed that she should be admitted to a nursing home for terminal care. This was arranged and until June 1972 she remained in bed in an expensive nursing home with her pain controlled with four-hourly injections of diamorphine and pethidine between doses if required.

21 June 1972. Mrs. M. was transferred to another home for financial reasons. Here she was reassessed by a consultant who specialized in rehabilitation for cancer patients. He studied all the previous X-rays and thoroughly examined the patient and gave his opinion that there was no evidence to prevent active mobilization with a view to discharge home.

22 June 1972. Mrs. M. was noted to be cheerful and enthusiastic at the prospect of getting up and walking.

On examination. Upper limbs were of normal strength. In the lower limbs there was full movement in all joints but all muscle groups had reduced tone. Although the muscle power was reduced it was remarkable that after almost twelve months in bed Mrs. M. was still able to 'straight leg raise'.

A spinal support had been worn prior to the admission one year previously.

Aims of treatment. (1) As pain did not appear to be a problem, the nursing staff were asked to wean Mrs. M. from the diamorphine and pethidine as directed by the house doctor.

(2) All muscle groups were to be strengthened.

(3) Balance and postural sense were to be re-educated.

(4) Walking re-education to be started as soon as possible.

(5) Mrs. M. was to be made as independent and self-reliant as possible within her limitations.

Plan of treatment. (1) Intensive bed exercises including slings and springs for quadriceps and gluteal muscle groups.

(2) Exercises for the intrinsic muscles of the feet were given with the patient sitting over the side of the bed with feet on a hard stool. The postural reflex was thus also stimulated through the feeling of a hard surface on the soles of the feet.

(3) Balance exercises were given while she was sitting over the side of the bed.

After three days, Mrs. M. was so anxious to try standing, that progression was made and she stood with the help of two people. Whilst standing, she was encouraged to mark time on the spot and then to take three steps to a chair.

26 June 1972. Mrs. M. had spent the whole weekend practising not only her exercises, but admitted taking a walk across the ward with the nurses! She was obviously well enough to come to the physiotherapy department and partake in a full programme of activities with other patients. Walking was commenced between parellel bars and progressed very rapidly to using one stick. She complained of pain in the region of the anterior superior iliac spine but on examination all movements were full, free and painless. She was strongly reassured.

30 June 1972. Mrs. M. went home for the weekend and was delighted to find she could potter around her own home again.

She had been advised not to be too active on this first visit.

10 July 1972. Mrs. M. was now fully ambulant and was able to manage stairs. She had complained of acute pain in the right ribs and had been X-rayed. No deposits or fracture were noted. The consultant deputed the physiotherapist to explain and reassure Mrs. M. that following prolonged bed rest she must expect aches and pains, but at the same time she must not imagine that every pain meant a recurrence of disease. This is a clear example of an established three-way relationship between surgeon, physiotherapist and patient, as well as illustrating the now oft-quoted adage of making time, sitting down, listening and explaining.

26 July 1972. Mrs. M. was discharged home and followed up at monthly intervals.

November 1972. Mrs. M. was very well and the consultant noted 'Does her own cooking and takes care of her children and husband. Can do her shopping and looks extremely well'.

It is possible to record that Mrs. M. remained at home until June 1973 when she required further irradiation to a deposit in the ilium. During September and October 1973 she received treatment for a severe anaemia but subsequently she improved and again returned home. She died in the autumn of 1974.

Relief of pain

Pain is defined as an unpleasant or distressing sensation due to bodily injury or disorder. Many people today still think in terms of cancer causing pain. This general thought is not true, though some cancers will cause physical pain. Nowadays, thanks to the work of Dr. Cicely Saunders and others, the control of pain by means of the skilful use of drugs is better understood and there should be no reason why any patient should be allowed to suffer pain.

Physical pain in cancer patients may be caused by: (1) pressure of a primary tumour upon nerves or pain-producing areas; (2) metastases of the vertebral bodies causing collapse and consequent pressure on the spinal nerves; (3) fibrosis following irradiation for treatment of a tumour; (4) a tumour which engulfs a nerve plexus.

Pain is seldom a feature of an early cancer. Relief of physical pain can be by medical means, i.e. drugs, or by surgical intervention, or in the case of some bone metastases, by irradiation.

SURGICAL METHODS

(1) Removal of the tumour.
(2) Decompression of the spinal cord.
(3) Drainage of fluid, e.g. abdominal paracentesis.
(4) Chordotomy or rhizotomy.
(5) Nerve blocking.

The first three of the above methods are self-explanatory. Chordotomy and rhizotomy are procedures which are resorted to only in very intractable cases, but the last method, nerve blocking, is quite frequently used and the physiotherapist may well become involved.

Nerve blocking is mostly used for intractable pain involving the sacral and lower lumbar roots, which occurs mostly in patients with cancer of the bladder, uterus or rectum. A local anaesthetic injection will give an indication as to how effective a block would be. Intrathecal alcohol or phenol are the blocking agents usually tried (Robbie, 1969), and the method of administration is well described by Markham (1970).

Following such injections there may be loss of control of bowel or bladder (if an ileal bladder or colostomy is established, this side-effect will not matter); there may also be numbness or weakness and difficulty in walking (Robbie, 1971).

Physiotherapy treatment. Many patients who have nerve blocking are active and working and therefore must be rehabilitated to walking and independence. It is the numbness which probably is the most disabling side-effect. Frenkel's exercises help to re-establish positional sense and patients can progress from doing them in a sitting position to performing them walking between parallel bars. The use of a stick when walking is fully justified for such patients, if for no other reason than a boost to morale! The numbness is seldom so severe as to make for a serious disability and the fact that the pain is relieved is sufficient for patients to accept a minor annoyance. Adequate pre-blocking explanation by the doctor is imperative and patients must clearly understand the possibility of side-effects.

OTHER ASPECTS OF PAIN

Any physical pain is intensified by mental anguish, and if the latter can be assuaged, the physical pain can become tolerable. Many of these patients can be helped by the physiotherapist who applies sound commonsense, compassion and understanding together with a love of life.

General classwork and suitable games with other patients will help, and an encouragement to think of other people and indeed lend a helping hand for some other patient in the ward, will also help towards a better acceptance of controllable pain. Everyone's pain tolerance is different, and a physiotherapist can sometimes help the doctor in assessing the degree of pain which a particular patient may have. Here again classwork can be most revealing! Other patients can often help the frightened patient in a way not possible for the professional.

Mental pain can be as disabling as physical pain and requires skilled counselling as well as the right use of tranquillizers or stimulants. The physiotherapist's part must be as a listener and here massage may be of immense help. To some patients such a 'ministry of touch' can provide the greatest help and offer an outlet for seeking additional help. If massage is requested the physiotherapist should not feel that she is being used as a 'makeshift' or as a 'last hope', but should accept the request as a real challenge to provide the help that is probably desperately required.

Chapter Twelve: The role of the physiotherapist in public education concerning cancer

Great strides have been made in the treatment of cancer. Prevention must, however, be the real goal of those who work in this field, and the prevention of cancer really involves education and an understanding of the disease.

The overall aim of public education should be to create by all ethical means a climate of opinion that is both informed and vigilant and not dominated by exaggerated fears. Without loss of truth, stress needs to be laid on the optimistic and little-known aspects of cancer, and which now get lost in the maelstrom of gloomy gossip about those who have not responded to treatment and the ghastly despondent emphasis which is placed on the annual mortality lists.

Prudence bids us accept that this will be a long process, conditioned as we have been to the centuries of hopelessness which have characterized the teaching on cancer. Into this long-term educational project must come those physiotherapists who are most involved in the care and treatment of cancer patients, and particularly those who work in the specialized oncological centres and radiotherapy units.

Education must be a two-way process for we must first educate ourselves before we can disseminate knowledge to others. There are, it is suggested, three main ways in which this knowledge may be acquired: by reading, questions and observations, and all these should be second nature to the physiotherapist.

READING

General background reading about the disease is essential, and the reader is referred to a selected list of suitable books (see p. 195). From time to time a survey of relevant literature is necessary, and the author recommends everyone to make friends with the librarian at the hospital medical library.

Then there is the reading of patients' notes, which can contain a wealth of information if rightly used. Look at the occupation: has the patient been at risk? e.g. the man who becomes paralysed from a bony secondary from a bladder cancer may well have worked in the rubber industry. Look at the family history: the young woman with a breast cancer may have had a mother, grandmother or sister with the same condition, and so one learns that sometimes breast cancer runs in a family and that such high-risk families should be screened regularly. Gradually these pieces of information grow, until at last a picture begins to take shape. This kind of knowledge will be added to through the years and indeed will never be complete.

Then there is 'light reading', the popular weeklies and monthlies which point to the latest cures, or highlight the common cancer operations, e.g. mastectomy, colostomy or laryngectomy, or describe some sensational diet or drug. Those of us who work with cancer patients know only too well the problems and difficulties which can result from such articles. Patients will ask our opinion of such writings and sensible answers based on known facts must be given. In dealing with cancer patients there can be no substitute for proper professional advice and physiotherapists should not hesitate to give such advice.

QUESTIONS

Attendance on ward rounds, clinics and seminars all give opportunity to ask questions relating to specific patients or conditions or to ask about cancer generally. All through this work the need for establishing a good relationship with the consultant has been stressed and this too will allow opportunity to ask for explanations and to discuss new ideas.

OBSERVATION

The reaction of patients to their condition, their treatment and their recovery should be noted. Textbooks can only give an academic and theoretical assessment of situations; observation will give the practical assessment. Every patient is an individual and no attempt should ever be made to neatly slot him into a type. Observation through follow-up of patients will enable one to realize how well many of them are over many years. The author has watched some patients now for over fifteen years and has found it fascinating to see how their reactions and those of the family have fluctuated.

Observation, too, is necessary to find out about facilities in the locality for early diagnosis, as well as general services available for cancer patients.

These are fundamental methods of acquiring knowledge that should enable any physiotherapist to establish a sound background of information which she is then able to impart to the lay public and also to her colleagues and other professionals.

The disseminating of knowledge

Any opportunity which presents itself should be seized upon to educate, whether it is only one individual or a group.

Patients often find it easier to communicate with a nurse or paramedical professional rather than a doctor, and the physiotherapist could well be the person to whom a frightened lady confides, 'I have found a lump in my breast, what should I do?' This is your chance to reassure at once that most breast lumps are benign but that they must be examined as soon as possible. The patient may be willing to go to her own doctor, but many are afraid of bothering their doctors with what they consider to be trifles. Such a response calls for firmness and the assurance that they will not be wasting a doctor's time. It may be that there are special facilities available in the locality and the physiotherapist can direct the patient there, even to the point of offering to come with her or ringing up and making the appointment. This *is* education in the practical manner tempered with sympathy and understanding.

Then there are the women who ask about cervical smears, who can be directed to Family Planning Clinics or the cervical screening clinics which are held by most local authorities. It is quite a good idea to collect the addresses of such services in a given locality and keep them pinned on the department notice-board.

Patients will also express their fears and this is where one should be able to discuss the specific question with kindly authority. Try not to talk about cures, but rather talk in terms of survival times; always show a positive approach and aim to encourage anyone to go to a doctor at once if they have symptoms which do not clear up. If one talks in terms of survival one can also impress on the patient that this will be better if an early diagnosis is made.

If a patient asks for advice and help, follow it up and make sure that the problem has been resolved. There is also so much dangerous nonsense talked that requires firm positive denial. The physiotherapist with a good background of simple facts and understanding can do much to counteract this and yet keep a person's respect.

As well as talking, there is education by example and here one must cite smoking! Whether physiotherapists are smokers or non-smokers themselves, there should be the simple rule of *no smoking* in all physiotherapy departments and staffrooms.

Lastly, education comes from the ability to speak from one's own experience through treating patients. In all education on the cancer subject, it is right to remember that, basically, people are frightened when they hear the word mentioned. It therefore obtains that reassurance and cautious optimism are as important as the imparting of factual knowledge and this can be confidently offered if you have had experience with patients.

The Cancer Information Association at Oxford issues a list of questions and answers for nurses which could be useful to physiotherapists. It enumerates the most common queries and gives short, simple explanations.

Each person will work out her own method of education and dissemination of knowledge. The author puts example at the top, with listening to patients' worries and the offering of a practical answer as a close second, and preventive education as such at the bottom. Others will certainly not agree, but 'soapbox' exhortation to do this, that or the other, or not to do it as the case may be, can have the opposite effect to what is intended. Life has to be lived and there is no purpose in making it more difficult, but equally one can point the way to a better understanding of the disease by stressing a simple, practical, helpful code.

Physiotherapists are essentially practical people and could be well suited to such an approach. The antidote to fear and uncertainty is always positive reassurance and practical help to solve the uncertainty.

A comprehensive list of organizations concerned with research, information and welfare for cancer patients is appended (see p. 197). In hospitals it is the responsibility of the Social Service Department to provide such information, but one is often asked about these matters by people elsewhere and it is useful to have some idea of available services in given localities. Almost all the research and information services will send full details of their work on request. Admission to the various Homes is either via the hospital or through the general practitioner direct to the Home.

'Knowledge is the antidote of Fear', wrote Emerson, and that could well be the motto for all of us who work with cancer patients.

Chapter Thirteen: **Nutrition and the rehabilitation of the cancer patient** by J. W. T. Dickerson, Ph.D. (Cantab.), F.I.Biol, Professor of Human Nutrition, University of Surrey and Jackie Tredger, B.Sc. (Surrey), S.R.D., Lecturer in Dietetics, University of Surrey

Introduction

Many illnesses, or accidents, occur in otherwise well-nourished individuals, and do not, generally speaking, result in any grave nutritional problems. We know, from the work initiated in Glasgow about 40 years ago by Sir David Cuthbertson, that trauma and surgical operations result in a change in the metabolism of the body so that tissue, mainly skeletal muscle, is catabolised, and there is an increase in the amounts of nitrogen, potassium, phosphorus and sulphur excreted in the urine. Whilst some of this breakdown of tissue is the result of postoperative starvation, there is also superimposed on this, the result of the metabolic disturbances caused by the injury itself, and partly mediated by the steroid hormones secreted by the adrenal glands. Well-nourished individuals are well able to survive these combined catabolic changes, and derive the energy for life and the material for the healing of their wounds from their own resources.

The patient with cancer may present quite a different problem. Tumours may grow slowly, and their presence be often unsuspected, until they cause discomfort or interfere with appetite or food intake. Anorexia may also result from worry and anxiety about a known or suspected tumour. Loss of weight may then be a major and continuing problem. Furthermore, the treatment of cancer may involve radical surgery alone, or in combination, with radiation and drug therapy, and we shall consider the nutritional problems that may be associated with these treatments and the ways by which attempts may be made to rectify them.

It is very important to appreciate that the care of a patient with cancer and his, or her, restoration to the best possible measure of health is a team effort, and that although there are those with particular knowledge and expertise in certain aspects of care, full benefit is only derived by the patient when there is understanding and appreciation of an inter-disciplinary nature. The physiotherapist may not feel competent to give detailed nutritional advice, but she should at least be aware of the kind of problems that her patients are likely to have, and be able to appreciate the contribution that a colleague may be able to make. Oftentimes, it will be found that the advice necessary is simple, and the psychological value of this when given with 'authority' should not be underestimated.

Nutritional problems found in the patient with cancer

1. WEIGHT LOSS

A fall in body weight is not an invariable occurrence in a patient with cancer, but in some cases it is the sign that makes the patient seek medical advice. By far the most common cause of weight loss is a diminished intake of food. The energy entering the body is less than the basal energy of metabolism and the energy cost of the various activities involved in living. Indeed, in the patient with cancer the energy requirement may well be somewhat higher than that of a normal person of the same sex, and of similar age and activity.

In certain situations tumours may mechanically interfere with the amount of food that can be taken. This occurs, for instance, with carcinoma of the oesophagus when the swallowing of solid food is partially, or even totally, prevented, and because of this the patient will take only fluids. Often in patients with carcinoma of the stomach the tumour produces a feeling of 'fullness' with consequent loss of appetite, reduced food intake and hence loss of body weight. It is now almost 40 years since it was first suggested that some tumours produce one or more 'toxohormones' which accelerate tissue catabolism. Analgesic and sedative drugs may also result in a loss of appetite and reduction in food intake. Malabsorption may be a factor in some cases.

The fall in body weight is initially accounted for by the mobilization and metabolism of body fat (Watkin, 1959). Chronic malnutrition, however, causes a reduction in cell mass, particularly as the result of catabolism of muscle tissue. If the patient has been confined to bed for any length of time, this will, of itself cause an increased excretion of nitrogen in the urine, and also after a lapse of time, increases in the excretion of calcium and phosphate (Dietrick et al., 1948), thus showing that not only muscle, but also the skeleton is involved.

It is desirable to nutritionally rehabilitate the patient before treatment, if this is possible as it may well reduce the period of convalescence. The restoration of body tissue however, is time consuming and the clinician finds himself in somewhat of a dilemma if surgery cannot be delayed. It may then be considered more important to treat the patient and postpone the nutritional rehabilitation until afterwards.

2. EFFECTS OF TREATMENT

(1) SURGERY

We have already referred to the metabolic effects of surgery. The magnitude of these effects depends on the nutritional state of the patient for the response of a well-nourished person is greater than that of a malnourished one. The effects also increase with the severity of the surgery. The surgical removal of tumours often necessitates considerable sacrifice of neighbouring tissues in order to reduce the possibility of spread of the tumour. Surgery on any part of the alimentary tract results in a disturbance of the patients' ability to consume, digest or absorb food. The nature and extent of the disturbance depends on the location and extent of the surgery.

Excision of tumours of the mouth or pharynx may make the patient dependent for a time upon tube-feeds and solid food may have to be permanently replaced by a 'soft' and semi-fluid diet. After oesophagectomy nutritional rehabilitation is a lengthy process, and the patient may only slowly return toward ideal body weight. If the tumour was at the lower end of the oesophagus and involving the cardia of the stomach, the more extensive oesophago-gastrectomy will probably have been performed. Reduction in size of the stomach, or its total excision, results in a loss of the 'hopper' function of the stomach so that consumption of anything like an adequate amount of food becomes a problem. Moreover, the acid normally secreted by the stomach facilitates the absorption of iron, and 50 per cent of the absorption of this mineral occurs in the duodenum. Iron deficiency anaemia is therefore a common complication of gastric operations, although it may not be manifest for 5 to 15 years postoperatively. Similarly, a gastric operation, and particularly, a total gastrectomy, interferes with the absorption of vitamin B_{12} due to a reduction in the secretion of the intrinsic factor. These patients then become dependent upon injections of vitamin B_{12} for the rest of their lives. Liver stores of the vitamin enable a previously well-nourished subject to survive for 3 to 5 years without the injections, but experience shows that it is all too easy for these supplements to be forgotten and the patient become unnecessarily debilitated.

Osteomalacia with generalized bone pains and diminished mineralization of the bones may occur in a proportion of gastrectomized patients. Osteoporosis with accompanying back pain due to vertebral collapse may also occur. Both these conditions may reflect a combination of a simple reduction in food intake and specific malabsorption defects. For example, the fat-soluble vitamins, including vitamin D, may be lost in excessive quantities if steatorrhoea is present. Again, these tend to be 'late' complications of gastric surgery, but ones that a physiotherapist may well meet, if not in a cancer patient, in one that has had a partial gastrectomy some years previously for a gastric ulcer.

The organs of the body have considerable powers of adaptation, and although diarrhoea for the first 2 to 3 months after total colectomy and ileorectal anastomosis, semi-formed tooth-paste-like stools are then formed which are voided two to four times per day. The problems of patients with a colostomy vary in severity with the position of the colostomy. Generally, however, these patients suffer from some diarrhoea. Nutritional maintenance and rehabilitation depends on obtaining a balance between reducing the diarrhoea and also the food residues presented for evacuation. A diet which is normal, but with a low residue may be necessary.

(II) RADIOTHERAPY

There is a moving account in the medical literature by a physician recounting her experiences following radiotherapy for cancer of the pharynx (MacCarthy-Leventhal, 1959) which serves to emphasize the profound psychological, physiological, and nutritional after-effects which may occur. Damage to taste-buds results in a condition described as 'mouth-blindness' which reduces food acceptance and leads to anorexia. In this condition all food becomes tasteless, and improper food preparation and presentation create a serious situation since 'the patients are not hungry anyway, and it is easier to starve'. The food is tasteless and must therefore be served in such a way as to make use of its aroma as a stimulus to appetite.

This condition may result in different problems in different patients, and this is illustrated by the following case history, which incidentally also illustrates the value of a physiotherapist appreciating the importance of nutritional problems and recommending the patient to seek appropriate advice. In other words, it is an example of the 'team approach' to the rehabilitation of the cancer patient. 'B' was a married man in his early sixties who had had a partial glossectomy for cancer of the tongue with follow-up radiotherapy. His taste-buds were partially destroyed with the result that all food tasted 'bitter' and intake was reduced to egg-flips, some wine and spirits and a considerable amount of beer. His wife became very concerned, particularly as the local general practitioner was convinced that 'B' was an alcoholic and required psychiatric treatment.

At this point a physiotherapist was contacted in desperation about the possibility of rehabilitation. She recognized the gravity of the nutritional problem and referred the patient for advice. When visited, the patient was found in a thoroughly dejected condition, somewhat confused and emaciated. Apart from the general lack of food, it seemed likely that the condition was in considerable measure due to a deficiency of thiamin which had induced a downwardly directed spiral of progressive depletion and general malnutrition. With the help of his wife, 'B' was persuaded to stop drinking spirits and greatly reduce his consumption of beer. At the same time a somewhat bland food composed of 'Prosol' (Unigate), Caloreen and milk was prescribed together with substantial doses of a multivitamin preparation. Improvement was dramatic and within two weeks the patient had regained some weight, had much more energy and a will to live. Within a further three weeks he was sufficiently improved to be spending two or three hours in his garden and making plans to sell his house and emigrate.

The small and large bowel are damaged in a small but significant number of patients receiving radiotherapy for abdominal cancer. The intestinal mucosa is second only to bone marrow in its sensitivity to radiation due to the normally short half-life of its cells. Altered intestinal function may well occur at the time of therapy, but in the majority of cases normal function is restored. In some patients, however, symptoms may recur after an interval of a year or more. There may be diarrhoea, obstruction or fistula formation. The latter may necessitate bowel resection which reduces the absorptive surface, and may increase the diarrhoea and malabsorption. Close follow-up of these patients is necessary in order to prevent them becoming 'nutritional cripples'. Any patient with persistent loss of appetite should be referred to a nutritionist.

(III) CHEMOTHERAPY

Hormones, and particularly adrenocorticoid steroids, may cause disturbances of nutrition. Losses of nitrogen, calcium and potassium may occur, and the magnitude of the losses depends upon the type of steroid, the dosage and the duration of treatment.

It must be remembered that most of the chemotherapeutic agents affect normal cells as well as cancer cells. It follows, therefore, that, as with radiotherapy, those cells which are normally multiplying at the age of the patient will be affected by the drug. In the adult this includes the mucosal cells of the intestine, blood-forming cells, the cells of hair follicles and the squamous epithelial cells of the skin. From the point of view of nutrition, effects on the intestine are the most important since they may well result in malabsorption of nutrients. The magnitude of these effects will depend on the nature of the drug, dosage, duration of treatment, changes in rates of excretion or metabolism and also upon individual susceptibility. The nutritional status of the patient will be one factor involved in individual susceptibility because, generally speaking, better nourished patients are able to withstand higher doses of drugs (Shils, 1974). Nutrition also affects the rates at which drugs are metabolized (Basu and Dickerson, 1974) and hence again their toxicity.

Folic acid plays an important role in the synthesis of DNA and thus antimetabolites of folic acid, such as methotrexate, reduce DNA synthesis and cell multiplication. These substances cause changes in the small intestine and hence reduce the rate of absorption of xylose and presumably of nutrients.

The fluorinated pyrimidones markedly affect the gastro-intestinal mucosa. In patients receiving 5-fluorouracil the bone marrow may become megaloblastic and show changes similar to those found in pernicious and other megaloblastic anaemias due to nutritional deficiencies. Some patients also show biochemical evidence of thiamine deficiency (Basu et al., 1974).

A summary of the effects of the different drugs used in chemotherapy is given in Table I. All the drugs listed cause nausea and vomiting and depend for their cytotoxic action upon their toxicity. Most of the drugs also cause anorexia, and diarrhoea and stomatitis are also common effects.

Table I Drugs used in chemotherapy and their effects (adapted from Hegedus and Pelham, 1975)

Type	Drugs	Stomatitis	Anorexia	Toxicity Vomiting	Nausea	Diarrhoea	Other effects
Alkylating agents	Cyclophosphamide		×	×	×		Oral ulcerations
	Melphalan			×	×		
	Nitrogen mustard		×	×	×		Metallic taste in mouth following injection, headache, fever
Antibiotics	Actinomycin D	×	×	×	×	×	Oral ulcerations
	Bleomycin	×	×	×	×		Fever, pulmonary toxicity
	Doxorubicin	×		×	×	×	Cardiac toxicity, red urine
Antimetabolites	Cytarabine		×	×	×	×	Oral inflammation and/or ulcerations, abdominal pain
	5-Fluorouracil	×	×	×	×	×	Oral ulcerations
	Hydroxyurea	×	×	×	×	×	Constipation, ulceration of buccal mucosa, renal dysfunction
	6-Mercaptopurine		×	×	×		Fever, liver dysfunction
	Methotrexate	×	×	×	×	×	Hepatic toxicity, oral ulcerations, gingivitis
Vinca alkaloids	Vinblastine	×	×	×		×	Constipation abdominal pain, glossitis, numbness in extremities
	Vincristine			×	×		Constipation, abdominal pain, numbness in extremities
Others	Nitrosoureas		×	×	×		Prolonged anorexia

3. CACHEXIA

Loss of body weight may occur in patients with cancer some time before there is any appreciable loss of appetite and decrease in food intake. It is now over a century since Pettenkofer and Voit reported that a patient with leukaemia had a higher than normal oxygen consumption and energy requirement which did not fall at night in the normal way. Subsequent studies on patients with different kinds of oncological disease have confirmed this original observation, and it seems clear that the metabolic rate varies directly with the activity of the disease. It is impossible to generalize about the magnitude of this effect, but there is one report (Waterhouse et al., 1951) of a patient being in negative energy balance on an intake of 2,700 kcal (11·3 MJ), the balance not becoming positive until the intake was 3,255 kcal (13·6 MJ).

The energy requirement in excess of that derived from the diet is made available from the body's own fat stores. In advanced disease where the intake of protein may be insufficient to meet the tumour's requirements for amino acids, body protein will be broken down and albumen, in particular, is metabolized. A tumour has, in fact, been likened to a 'nitrogen trap' (Waterhouse et al., 1951) building its own substance from amino acids liberated from the tissues of the host. Anaemia is also commonly found in the cancer patient.

It is not difficult to visualize the development of a vicious circle in which the tumour, worry and anorexia all act in cyclical fashion to reduce the mass and vitality of the patient. Fortunately, cachexia is not now a common finding, and there is little doubt that it can be prevented. The vigour with which the nutritional rehabilitation of such patients is attempted will depend on the prognosis that may reasonably be expected. There may well be no merit in simply keeping the patient alive, what has been called 'medicated survival' (Vickery, 1974). However, where life of some quality is still possible there is no excuse for not attempting to prevent the development of cachexia. There is one report (Pereira et al., 1955) of bedfast patients in a hospital for terminal care being restored to their families as a result of aggressive nutritional rehabilitation achieved initially with the aid of tube feeding (*vide infra*).

Psychological aspects of nutrition in rehabilitation

The patient with cancer may have little or no appetite, be emaciated and in a poor psychological state. The importance of the patient's state of mind cannot be too strongly emphasized for, even in well-nourished people, psychological upsets lead to poor utilization of food (Widdowson, 1951). The food itself must be highly nutritious with a high content of energy, protein, vitamins and minerals and of the smallest possible bulk. Turner (1966) noted the frequency with which simply the removal to hospital, and the frequent provision of small meals attractively prepared and presented, results in an almost immediate improvement of the patient's appetite. The chain of factors producing anorexia may well be broken by reassurance and freedom from responsibility.

Food may be good and highly nutritious, but unless it is eaten it will not benefit the patient. This underlines the importance, where it is possible to do so, of talking to the patient about his food and finding out likes and dislikes. Furthermore, expectancy of receiving food that is particularly liked may help to promote a failing appetite. In addition, it is necessary to pay considerable attention to the texture, appearance, and, if possible, the aroma of a meal. Ulceration of the mouth, whether as a result of radiotherapy or chemotherapy necessitates the provision of a non-irritant diet of a consistency suited to the patients' ability to chew and swallow. Bland diets of this kind all too often appear uninteresting, and some attempt should be made to include at least one coloured item of food on the plate. If food has to be reduced to a soft consistency this is best done either by the patient, or if this is not possible, in sight of the patient, so that again there is opportunity for the appetite to be stimulated. Where there is little sense of taste as much use should be made as possible of hot dishes that have an appetizing aroma.

Special diets

1. SUPPLEMENTED ORAL INTAKE

Oral feeding is always the method of choice, and every effort should be made to increase the nutrient intake of patients with poor appetites. This may involve offering one of a variety of palatable low bulk supplements now available. These include Complan and Carnation Instant Breakfast Food. Alternatively it may be sufficient to use skimmed milk powder or eggs for fortification of the usual diet. However, in some patients this must be complemented, or replaced entirely, by other forms. It is very important that an assessment of the patient's nutritional state be made, and if adequate food cannot be taken orally steps taken to institute another form of nourishing the patient. The physiotherapist may well play a role here in encouraging reluctant clinicians to pass a naso-gastric tube or put up an intravenous drip. Delay may well reduce the patient's chances of recovery, or make rehabilitation more difficult or extended.

2. TUBE-FEEDING

Patients who because of loss of appetite fail to eat sufficient food to maintain or regain their body weight may be fed conveniently through a naso-gastric tube. This route of food administration is also useful for those patients in whom swallowing is painful or difficult. It should be seen as a means of nutritional rehabilitation in its own right with specific indications and not as an easy alternative to parenteral nutrition. In fact, in order for it to be successful in patients with metabolic disturbances, there must be the same attention to detail in the composition of the tube-feed as that given parenteral nutrition.

The simplest form of tube-feed is prepared by blending puréed and liquid foods. Real foods are preferable as these will have odours which are psychologically important for the patient. A breakfast feed of strained cereals, egg, glucose or Gastro-caloreen, oil and milk may be followed at noon and in the evening by liquidized meals of good nutritional quality. Tea, coffee, or alternative drinks should be served to the patient in a recognizable fashion. If as many normal foods as possible are used it should be possible to avoid nutritional deficiencies. Foods that may be included in these diets, as indeed for those for normal oral consumption, will be governed by a knowledge of those that can be tolerated. Thus, ordinary milk must be excluded if the lactose cannot be tolerated. Similarly, in patients with steatorrhoea the fat content of the diet must be reduced or replaced by medium chain triglycerides (MCT oil). The latter are very useful as they have the same energy value as normal fat (triglyceride) but are absorbed much more easily (see Senior, 1968).

This kind of feed is only a little more expensive than a normal diet, but it is often difficult to meet the patient's requirements in a volume of feed that can be tolerated. An alternative feed can be based on Complan, Gastro-caloreen, milk and MCT oil with added vitamins. With these as the main constituents it is easy to calculate the protein, energy, mineral and vitamin intake. Special attention must be paid to the latter and supplements in the form of syrups added to the feed. In formulating these feeds, it should be remembered that the protein intake should be 60 g per day or more for a patient with normal renal function, and that for optimal utilization it will be necessary to supply energy at the rate of 200 kcal (0·84 MJ), per gram of nitrogen. Feeds of this kind will produce diarrhoea unless they are suitably diluted, and as a rule they should contain one kcal per ml of feed.

A further kind of tube-feed that may be used is the 'elemental diet'. The name implies that all the constituent components are known. They are useful for patients in whom the secretion of digestive enzymes is reduced, and those in whom the absorptive surface of the small intestine is reduced or damaged. They are designed to present nutrients to the intestinal mucosa in the most readily absorbable form. The nitrogen in them is present in the form of amino acids and for this reason the solutions have an unpleasant taste. Since they can be taken orally, the taste is usually disguised by the addition of acceptable flavours. A number of these diets are now available, but they should be used only for patients with malabsorption. A comparison of the comparative costs of the different types of tube-feeds shows that 90 g protein and 2,600 kcal (10·9 MJ), can be provided in a mixture of Complan and Caloreen for £0·40 per day whereas provision of 40 g protein and 1800 kcal (7·56 MJ) as Vivonex (an 'elemental' tube feed) costs £5·00 per day (Fowell et al., 1977).

Unpleasant side-effects to tube-feeding are very often not due to the composition of the feed, but to its mode of administration. It must be remembered that a previously malnourished patient cannot be expected suddenly to tolerate a full feed in one day without side-effects. The strength of the feeds must be increased gradually over a few days. It is also important that the feeds themselves should be at room temperature. It is also not uncommon for a nurse to be seen holding a large syringe full of feed in a towel because it is too hot, and with determination pushing the feed down a nasogastric tube! The angle of the feed is also important and nurses have been observed feeding recumbent patients through a tube with the foot of the bed raised on blocks (Jones, 1975).

In conscious patients a flexible, radio-opaque tube of internal diameter 1 mm (Baretex R2) is the ideal choice, and this may be passed into the stomach with the aid of a Saldinger wire. These thin tubes, in contrast to the more cumbersome Ryles tubes, have the advantage that they can be kept in position for many weeks without discomfort. The feed must, however, be made up with an appropriate consistency.

3. PARENTERAL FEEDING

Total parenteral nutrition (TPN) involves the provision of the patient's complete nutritional requirements by the intravenous route. Its use should be considered in circumstances where oral or tube feeding are contra-indicated and where prolonged maintenance or improvement in nutritional status will assist in recovery of the patient or permit significant palliation of an underlying disease. This form of nutrition may be life-saving in a variety of clinical situations—those pertinent to the cancer patient are shown in Table II.

Traditionally, many patients receive as parenteral nutrition three litres of dextrose saline per twenty four hours. This supplies a mere 575 kcal (2·4 MJ) and no nitrogen or trace elements. This may be suitable as short term parenteral support, but cannot be considered as adequate total parenteral nutrition. There are now available a wide variety of energy and nitrogen source solutions with which TPN regimens may be designed. The efficiency of these solutions has been well tested and they have been shown to be free of toxic effects.

Nitrogen source solutions are available as protein hydrolysates or synthetic crystalline amino acid solutions. The latter have the advantage of being specifically formulated and free of ammonia, but in practice do not have a better effect on nitrogen balance in adults than the protein hydrolysates (Tweedle et al., 1972).

In order for nitrogen sources to be fully utilized, adequate supplies of energy must be given simultaneously or shortly before. As with tube-feeds, administration of 200 kcal (0·84 MJ) is required for the optimum utilization of one gram of nitrogen (Lee 1974). Suitable energy sources for TPN include sugars, alcohol and fat emulsions. They may be used singly or in combination. Glucose is most certainly the carbohydrate of choice, being a normal physiological substrate, but fructose can be substituted in most situations.

Ethanol is a useful and pleasant energy source and may be safely used up to a dose of 1·5 g/kg body weight/24 hours without risk of intoxication (Lee, 1974).

Fat emulsions are particularly useful because they supply energy in a concentrated isotonic solution with virtually no osmotic effect. The provision of a comparable amount of energy in an equal volume of carbohydrate solution would require a solution with a hypertonicity which would tend to cause vein irritation and thrombophlebitis, see Table III. Fat emulsions are prepared from either cotton seed oil or soya bean oil, but only the latter should be used in long term parenteral feeding.

Requirements for fluid, electrolytes, vitamins and minerals will vary according to the patient's condition so that continual monitoring is essential. Basic requirements are frequently increased

Table II Possible indications for TPN in the cancer patient

Disorders of the gastro-intestinal tract	Obstruction of the oesophagus or stomach; malignant bowel disease.
Pre-operative feeding	Particularly in cases of carcinoma of the oesophagus or stomach when the patient requiring surgery is in a malnourished state.
Postoperative feeding	When return to a nutritionally adequate oral intake is likely to be delayed. When malabsorption may be a problem in the short or long term, e.g. after gastrectomy or massive bowel resection.
Adjunct to chemotherapy and radiotherapy	Anorexia and malabsorption are common side-effects. (See Table I.)

Table III Comparison of osmolality

	Osmolality mosm/kg	Energy kcal (MJ)
Plasma	300	
10% glucose	523	400 (1·68)
30% glucose	2,100	1,200 (5·04)
10% Intralipid (soya bean oil emulsion)	280	1,100 (4·62)

because of a pre-existing deficit or continuing abnormal losses. The regime must be planned having due regard to the predicted nutritional requirements of the patient.

There are two main routes of administration of parenteral nutrition—via a peripheral vein or central venous catheter. The peripheral route is ideal for short term nutritional support (less than one week), but due to the hypertonicity of the infused solutions there is a tendency to thrombophlebitis at the site of infusion. This may be reduced somewhat by changing the infusion site every 24–48 hours, but many chronically sick patients have a limited number of suitable veins. Patients requiring long term TPN are more appropriately treated by caval catheterization.

Total parenteral nutrition is now established as a safe and effective means of feeding patients unable to maintain normal alimentation. It was initially reserved for acutely ill patients in whom it was anticipated that normal nutrition would quickly be resumed but it is now used extensively for patients with severe chronic disorders requiring long term TPN. Indeed programmes have been developed which allow patients to carry out their TPN in their own home (Shils, 1975). Since malnutrition probably plays a major part in the death of most patients with malignant disease the contribution of TPN may be valuable to the quality, if not the quantity, of survival.

Special problems

1. THE NUTRITIONAL CRIPPLE

The increasing availability of a wide range of drugs, progress in anaesthesiology, and the development of methods for maintaining nutrition by the intravenous route or with elemental diets, have tempted surgeons to perform feats of resection which until recently were rejected because of their mortality or increased morbidity. However, 'while initial postoperative success using hyperalimentation (i.e. intravenous feeding) techniques has generated optimism, surgeons need to understand more fully the potential for long-term rehabilitation after specific procedures before subjecting both patients and their medical confrères, to whom they eventually transfer patient responsibility, to the experience of coping with a crippling disease without immediate cure and without immediate death' (Wright and Tilson, 1973).

Patients that have undergone massive gut resection whether for oncological or other disease are potentially cripples for the remainder of their lives. In the initial postoperative period they will require expert attention to all their nutritional requirements, including water and electrolytes. Should they survive these initial stages and achieve some measure of adaptation, they should then be referred to a nutritionist for continuing care. Patients that have had oesophago- and total gastrectomies benefit from periodic consultation even if these seem only to have a psychological effect. Advice on food choice, as well as reassurance about foods fancied, is often helpful.

2. SPECIFIC VITAMIN DEFICIENCIES

It is well-known that specific vitamin deficiencies affect the growth of tumours in experimental animals and it is becoming clear that in the human, tumours in certain sites may be associated with deficiencies of certain vitamins (Basu, 1977; Dickerson and Basu, 1977). Thus, patients with abdominal cancer have been found to have low blood levels of vitamin A. Low levels have also been found in the blood of patients with squamous and oat cell carcinoma of the lung, but not in those with large cell undifferentiated carcinoma. These latter findings do not prove that a low vitamin A status plays any role in the development of lung cancer, but it is of considerable interest in this connection that vitamin A inhibits the development of squamous metaplasia and squamous cell tumours in the respiratory tract of experimental animals.

There are some indications that the thiamine status of patients with breast cancer may be reduced as the tumour grows. In patients treated with the cytotoxic drug, 5-fluorouracil, thiamine status may be greatly reduced, possibly due to interference by the drug in the metabolism of the vitamin, and thiamin supplements may well be useful in the rehabilitation of such patients.

Vitamin C plays an important role in bone metabolism, and patients with skeletal metastases due to breast cancer have been found to have low concentrations of vitamin C in their blood, even though they were receiving a normally adequate intake. Furthermore, it has been suggested that high doses of vitamin C (5 g or more per day) may be useful in alleviating skeletal pain. This is an important suggestion for which there is some support in the literature.

Conclusions

It is quite clear that the patient with cancer may well be malnourished and that improvement of nutrition can play an important part in rehabilitation. Various means are available for doing this that can be adapted to the needs of the individual patient. There is no evidence whatever that malnutrition benefits the cancer patient, or that tumours grow faster in well-nourished individuals. The aim of rehabilitation is to improve as far as possible health and well-being, and thus the quality of the life that may remain. Nutritional rehabilitation would seem to be worthwhile even if it only restores sufficient vitality for the patient to leave hospital and end his life amongst those to whom he means most.

Acknowledgements

The senior author of this chapter, like the main author of this book, owes much to Mr. Ronald W. Raven for his interest and help, and most of all for sharing with us his great humanity. We are grateful to Mrs. Mary Lewis for so willingly undertaking the typing.

References

Basu, T. K. (1977). 'Significance of vitamins in cancer', *Oncology*. In Press.
Basu, T. K. and Dickerson, J. W. T. (1974). 'Inter-relationships of nutrition and the metabolism of drugs', *Chem-Biol. Interactions*, **8**, 193.
Basu, T. K., Dickerson, J. W. T., Raven, R. W. and Williams, D. C. (1974). 'The thiamine status of patients with cancer as determined by the red cell transketolase activity', *Internat. J. Vit. Nutr. Res.*, **44**, 53.
Deitrick, J. E., Whedon, G. D. and Shorr, E. (1948). 'Effects of immobilization upon various metabolic and physiologic functions of normal men', *Amer. J. Med.*, **4**, 3.
Dickerson, J. W. T. and Basu, T. K. (1977). 'Specific vitamin deficiencies and their significance in patients with cancer and receiving chemotherapy', *Nutrition and Cancer*. Ed. M. Winick, New York: Wiley. In Press.
Fowell, E., Lee, H. A. and Dickerson, J. W. T. (1977). 'Tube Feeding', *Nutrition in the Clinical Management of Disease*, Eds. J. W. T. Dickerson and H. A. Lee. London: Arnold.
Hegedus, S. and Pelham, M. (1975). 'Dietetics in a cancer hospital *Perspectives in Practice*, **67**, 235.
Jones, D. C. (1975). 'The Nutritional Nursing Care of Unconscious Patients in General Hospitals'. M.Phil. Thesis, University of Surrey.
Lee, H. A. (1974). 'The alcohols—ethanol, sorbitol, xylitol', *Parenta Nutrition in Acute Metabolic Illness*, Ed. H. A. Lee. London: Academic Press.
MacCarthy-Leventhal, E. M. (1959). 'Post-radiation mouth blindness', *Lancet*, **ii**, 1138.
Pereira, M. D., Conrad, E. J., Hicks, W. and Elman, R. (1955). 'Clinical response and changes in nitrogen balance, body weight, plasma proteins and hemoglobin following tube feeding in cancer cachexia', *Cancer*, **8**, 803.
Senior, J. R. (Ed.) (1968). *Medium Chain Triglycerides*. Philadelphia: Univ. of Pennsylvania Press.
Shils, M. E. (1974). 'Nutrition and neoplasia', *Modern Nutrition in Health and Disease*, 5th ed., p. 981. Eds. R. S. Goodhart and M. E. Shils. Philadelphia: Lea & Febiger.
Shils, M. E. (1975). 'A program for total parenteral nutrition at home', *Amer. J. Clin. Nutr.*, **28**, 1429.
Turner, C. M. (1966). 'The role of nutrition in the treatment of cancer' *Nutrition*, **20**, 60.

Tweedle, D. E. F., Spivey, J. and Johnston, I. D. A. (1972). 'The effect of four different amino acid solutions upon the nitrogen balance of postoperative patients', *Patenteral Nutrition*, Ed. A. W. Wilkinson. London: Churchill Livingstone.

Vickery, K. O. A. (1974). 'Medicated Survival—The Press, The Public, The Professions and the Patient', *Roy. Soc. Health, J.*, **94**, 118.

Waterhouse, C., Fenninger, L. D. and Keutmann, E. H. (1951). 'Nitrogen exchange and calorie expenditure in patients with malignant neoplasms', *Cancer*, **4**, 500.

Watkin, D. M. (1959). 'Increased fat utilization in the hypermetabolism of active neoplastic disease', *Acta Union Internationale Centre le Cancer*, **15**, 907.

Widdowson, E. M. (1951). 'Mental contentment and physical growth', *Lancet*, **i**, 1316.

Wright, H. K. and Tilson, M. D. (1973). *Post-operative Disorders of the Gastrointestinal Tract*. New York: Grune & Stratton.

Chapter Fourteen: **The psychological impact of cancer** by G. P. Maguire, M.R.C. Psych., Senior Lecturer in Psychiatry, The University Hospital of South Manchester

Introduction

Despite advances in the treatment of some cancers most people still view them as the commonest cause of death and the most alarming group of illnesses. Moreover, a fifth believe that they are never curable (Knopf 1974: Williams *et al.*, 1972).

As a consequence of this pessimism many of those who discover that they have cancer are likely to become very worried and frightened. The majority will be afraid that the cancer might spread through their bodies, cause endless pain and suffering, and lead to an early death.

Similarly, their close relatives will tend to assume that they will soon lose a loved one and wonder whether they will be able to cope with the strains of the illness and subsequent bereavement. They may also feel angry that all their hopes and plans will now be thwarted.

In addition to these general worries there may be more specific problems due to the types of treatment which are used. The treatments which are most likely to cause psychological difficulties include:

1. SURGERY

Which results in:
    (a) the loss and mutilation of important parts of the body; for example:

PSYCHOLOGICAL PROBLEMS

amputation of a breast (mastectomy)
amputation of a limb
head and neck surgery;
(b) the loss of internal organs which affect child-bearing functions and so may have particular emotional significance; for example:
loss of the womb (hysterectomy)
loss of ovaries (oophorectomy);
(c) the loss of normal body functions; for example:
loss of normal speech after laryngectomy
loss of ability to empty the bowels voluntarily after colostomy.

2. DRUG TREATMENTS

(a) *Chemotherapy*. The use of potent drugs such as methotrexate, cyclophosphamide, 6-mercaptopurine and vincristine to combat certain forms of cancer has become more widespread. Unfortunately these often cause severe vomiting, nausea, tiredness and hair loss as well as other unpleasant side-effects.

(b) *Hormones*. Some cancers, especially when they are more advanced, may be treated with oestrogens, androgens, progesterones or corticosteroids. Oestrogens may cause nausea and vomiting while testosterone can produce an unsightly increase in body hair, coarsening of the voice, and an increase in sex drive. Steroids often cause weight gain and may also precipitate serious psychiatric illness.

3. RADIOTHERAPY

Many patients associate having radiotherapy with a poor outcome. They may, therefore, become upset because of this and also because of the hair loss, fatigue, nausea and vomiting which can occur.

Both the general worries caused by cancers and the problems associated with particular treatments have to be coped with if the cancer patient and their families are to find life still worthwhile.

Unfortunately there is growing evidence that some of them fail to cope and develop serious psychological problems. The kind of problems that may arise will be discussed with particular reference to breast cancer.

The impact of breast cancer and mastectomy

DISCOVERY OF THE LUMP

Most women now know that a breast lump could turn out to be a cancer. In view of the prevailing pessimism about treatment it is not surprising that they can become very worried and frightened when they discover that they have a lump.

While their main fear is of cancer some women may be equally afraid of losing a breast. This fear will be especially intense when the bust has been important to the womens' sense of being attractive and valued both by themselves and others. It has been estimated that over 70 per cent of women will become preoccupied with one or both of these fears in the period before biopsy and that one in three will experience considerable distress (Chesser and Anderson 1975; Maguire 1976).

> When I found the lump, I just couldn't believe it. I'd only examined my breasts a month before and I'd found nothing. It was a terrible shock. My first thought was that it must be cancer. I mean you're bound to think that aren't you what with all the publicity there has been. Then I thought it might not be too advanced, even if it was cancer, because it hadn't been there when I last felt my breasts. But I just went to pieces over the next few days. I kept shouting to my husband and family that I didn't want to die. That I was still young. My husband called in our G.P. He gave me a sedative to calm me down.

Hence by the time they first attend a hospital clinic for examination of the breast lump many women are in a very worried frame of mind. They dread what might be said to them after the examination and history-taking have been completed. This distress is important because of the suffering that it causes and because it may prevent the women from registering accurately what is said to them by the surgeons or clinic staff.

Those women who are told unequivocally by the surgeon that their lump is benign and that further treatment is not needed will usually leave the clinic in a happier frame of mind. Those who are told that they will have to come into hospital for biopsy to determine the nature of the lump will continue to be distressed. The distress is likely to be greatest in those women who are going to turn out to have cancer. Examination of the ways in which surgeons communicate to women on their first visit to the clinic suggests that this is directly related to the fact that the surgeon is not able to use reassuring statements that the lump is probably going to be all right. Instead he is likely to have used phrases which indicate the possibility of cancer or euphemisms which strongly suggest it. An example of such a euphemism is: 'It could be a growth, but if it is it's not a very big one.'

As many as one in five of those women who are going to turn out to have cancer will experience moderately severe, or severe symptoms of anxiety (feeling on edge, headaches, sweating, palpitations) or depression (feeling low, weepy, lacking in energy, hopeless) in this interval of time between the clinic and admission.

> I just couldn't relax. It kept churning through my mind that it must be cancer. I couldn't get it out of my mind that he (the surgeon) had said it was a growth but not a big one. I mean when they say growth it must be cancer mustn't it. It was just like a nightmare. I felt ever so frightened and so very upset. I found I couldn't concentrate on anything and I kept bursting into tears. Every time anybody spoke to me I blew my top at them. Oh my poor husband. I don't know how he put up with me. I was in a shocking state. I felt I was no use to anyone like that and probably no use to them any more.

Unfortunately, only a quarter of those women who become distressed in the prebiopsy period usually make any mention of it to anyone connected with their care. Even when they do, for example, say 'I've been ever so worried since I found the lump', 'I've been on nerve pills since I found it', it is most unlikely that the surgeon or clinic staff will enquire directly about the reasons for this distress. It is more likely that they will make some general reassuring statement like 'don't worry, it will be all right, you are in good hands'. As a result, few of these distressed women will feel reassured by their visit. Some may be even more distressed than when they entered the clinic.

While only one in four women give verbal cues about their distress up to 70 per cent will give non-verbal cues. Thus they will look obviously anxious, weepy or very tense. Yet only rarely will the surgeon spot the worry and enquire about it. As a consequence, the treatment team will often seriously underestimate just how distressed many of these women are. Importantly, they will also miss the fact that some women have quite practical worries, for example who will look after the children when they come into hospital.

AFTER ADMISSION

For some women admission to hospital brings with it a great sense of relief.

> Once I got into hospital I felt much calmer. I was in such good hands. I thought that whatever I had they'd take good care of me and do the best they could. I knew they wouldn't let me down.

However, for other patients it meant a time of increasing fear because they knew that their period of uncertainty would soon be over and that they might have to face the fact that they did have cancer and could no longer kid themselves that they did not. This distress could sometimes be disabling for individual women as the following example illustrates:

> On the day I was admitted to hospital I was convinced that I had cancer. My mother had had a lump like mine. She had a terrible time. She died with it. I was terribly afraid that the

same thing would happen to me. When anyone came near me I kept asking them whether I had cancer or not. I think they got fed up with my asking but they just wouldn't say anything to me. They said I'd have to talk to the doctors about it. When sister came round to see me I tried to get her to tell me. I kept saying please tell me, I must know, I'm so sick with worry. She told me I was being a nuisance to her staff and should leave them alone and just pull myself together. I felt in a terrible state. I felt no one understood what I was feeling. There was nothing for it but to put my face to the pillow and just cry and cry. If only I could have really talked to someone about it I think it might have helped.

There is clearly a risk with the kind of patient who reacts in this frightened way that they may be labelled as difficult and uncooperative by the nursing and medical staff. Intense emotional distress is especially likely when, as in this patient, the women have known someone who died rather horribly from cancer. For it is obvious that they will predict that they will die in the same way.

Another way in which the womens' distress may be affected on admission to hospital is through their contact with patients who have been admitted previously but had a biopsy or mastectomy. This patient grapevine can clearly work in two ways. The women can either be given information that reassures them, for example that the procedure is not really very frightening and that they will soon feel well. On the other hand they may meet a woman who says it's a terrible experience and that it means they've got inoperable cancer.

AFTER SURGERY

How the women react to the discovery that they have lost a breast is related to the expectations they had before surgery and their level of emotional distress.

They will be particularly upset when they had not expected to lose a breast. Their optimism before surgery may, in some cases, have been reasonable in that it accorded with what the surgeons had told them. However, their optimism might also have represented their refusal to come to terms with evidence that their lump was serious in nature.

Another group who will also be disturbed by the breast loss will be those women who were particularly distressed before operation, either through fears of cancer or fears of mutilation.

> When I put my hand there I knew they'd taken it away. I was simply shattered. I felt so repulsive and deformed. How could I face the world feeling like this. Was there really any point in going on? I hit the depths that day. I'd never felt so low in all my life. I begged them not to let my husband in to see me. I thought he would just turn tail if he saw me like that. It really was the worst thing that has ever happened to me.

The women will also be much affected by the response of those around them. The nurse who is with them when they wake up after the operation or the physiotherapist who helps them with the exercises will often influence the way they feel, particularly their attitudes to their scars and disease.

In those instances where the woman cannot face the scar and actively avoids looking at it, it is likely that she will be even more reluctant to let her husband see it. This is usually because she believes that he will find her repulsive and will not want anything more to do with her. When the woman returns home she may suggest to her husband, as a way of avoiding him seeing the scar, that they sleep in separate beds because she still feels tired after the operation. If she is allowed to do this for some time it is quite likely that when they get together again their sexual relationship will have suffered considerably.

Some women are unable to tolerate their husbands suggesting love making because they are frightened of their reactions if they see them naked or caress them. These fears about the effects of the mutilation may be especially apparent in those women who are single or divorced. For they have the very real problem of how they can broach the fact that they've only got one breast to any new partner. They come to believe that there really is no hope for them.

Worries about their appearance can also be aggravated by any postoperative complications particularly swelling of the arm. They may take any swelling to mean that the cancer has not been eradicated or allow it to reinforce their views that they are now rather ugly, 'lopsided' or 'deformed'. The extent to which the women can be reassured that the cancer has been controlled and about their mutilation will determine how they adapt subsequently.

The importance of husbands being able to reassure their wives that they still love them is well illustrated in the following example.

> Every time I looked at it I thought my God how ugly—how can anyone bear me like this—I just didn't want to know about it—you know—sex anymore—but he kept at me. He told me it didn't make any difference. He'd rather have me with only one breast than not at all. I begged him to leave me alone, let me sleep alone—he got angry at me, told me not to be such a bloody fool—said he still loved me as much as always—looking back I'm sure that's what pulled me through.

The women can be much helped or hindered by the prostheses which they are given shortly after their discharge from hospital. Where the prosthesis is unsatisfactory, as it may be in up to a third of the women (Downie, 1976), this may cause women to avoid meeting people socially. For they may become convinced that people only need to look at them to tell that they've only got one breast and that they are so obviously misshapen. This kind of avoidance is particularly likely when it comes to buying new clothes or going to parties where they might be expected to wear relatively low-cut dresses or figure-clinging clothes. This problem of unsatisfactory prostheses is made worse by the fact that many of the women feel unable to complain about them or ask for a replacement.

The fear that the cancer might recur either in the other breast or in some other part of the body causes many women to be extremely sensitive to changes in their physical health. Headaches that would, before the operation, have been regarded as trivial and require at the most an aspirin, now become the sign of a possible tumour. Similarly aches and pains that would have been dismissed as just twinges may now cause the woman to believe that the cancer has spread to different parts of the body.

In the first few weeks after mastectomy the women may be given radiotherapy or chemotherapy. Since these treatments can cause unpleasant side-effects (see introduction) they may cause some women to become very upset (Maguire, 1976) or intensify the distress which they were experiencing already.

A study of the incidence of psychological problems in the first three to four months after mastectomy has confirmed that they can be considerable (Maguire, 1976).

Up to one in three of the women will have experienced moderately severe or severe symptoms of anxiety or depression. In some of the women these will have been so severe as to make them feel that life is not worth living and contemplate suicide. Major changes will also be evident in the sexual adjustment of some of the women. In over 40 per cent the women will have complained that they can no longer enjoy love-making as much as they could before operation and some will have completely ceased to have any sexual relationship with their husbands. In addition to these disturbances in their mood and sexual adjustment some of the women will also have experienced considerable difficulties in trying to cope with their day-to-day chores or work.

Follow-up twelve months after mastectomy shows that contrary to expectations many of the women will still be experiencing severe psychological problems. It is likely that one in five will be suffering from a depressive illness, one in six from an anxiety state, while a third will still be experiencing some difficulties in coping with their jobs. They will complain that they can only do the same job with considerable difficulty or have found it necessary to change their jobs either by a reduction in working hours or moving to a lighter job.

Unfortunately these various changes cannot be explained solely in terms of the progression of the breast cancer. For many of the women who cope least well and experience most depression and anxiety will be considered by the surgeons to have survived well from a physical point of view.

Thus, it must be expected that a small but important proportion of women who undergo mastectomy for breast cancer will experience quite serious emotional problems in the year after mastectomy.

Although there has been little study of how women adjust to mastectomy in the longer term the work that has been carried on at Kings' College Hospital in London suggests that these problems continue over several years (Greer, 1976).

PROBLEMS ASSOCIATION WITH RECURRENT OR ADVANCED BREAST DISEASE

Similarly, there has been little systematic study of the psychological effects of advanced or recurrent breast disease. However, it seems likely that the pattern of emotional difficulties will be the same as in the early stages.

The discovery that the cancer has recurred or is advancing will cause considerable shock and depression. Whether this depression continues will usually depend on how well the woman can come to terms with the knowledge that she may not have long to live. It will also depend on how confident she is that any pain, sickness or breathlessness will be adquately controlled by the care she receives, and whether she can come to terms with the loss of her role as mother, wife and possibly breadwinner in the family.

Her efforts to cope may be severely hampered by the treatments which she will receive for her advanced disease. Thus she may undergo surgery to remove her ovaries (oophorectomy), adrenal glands (adrenalectomy), or hypophysis (hypophysectomy).

Similarly, the hormones which may be given in advanced disease, (see introduction) may also produce unpleasant effects (Holland, 1973).

If women become unduly depressed or anxious as a result of these various treatments and their side-effects, this may have considerable repercussions on their management. For example, it may make them much more sensitive to pain and may make pain control extremely difficult without the use of very high doses of pain relieving drugs.

In view of these findings it seems likely that a similar range of problems will be found in other types of mutilating surgery such as head and neck surgery and limb amputation.

IMPACT OF COLOSTOMY FOR ANO-RECTAL CANCER

When a patient is given a permanent colostomy after surgery for ano-rectal cancer, he has to cope with several problems: worry that he might have had cancer and that it has not been completely removed; the presence of an appliance on the abdomen into which faeces will discharge periodically; impairment of the ability to have sexual intercourse; and management of the appliance. These problems are formidable and, as with mastectomy, it is now clear that a substantial number of patients will develop psychiatric problems (23 per cent) especially depressive illness (Devlin et al., 1971).

The effect on sexual adjustment may also be catastrophic. Over half of the men who have an abdomino-perineal resection followed by colostomy suffer a serious deterioration in their ability to have sexual intercourse and it is likely that women may experience similar difficulties, largely because the surgery may sever essential nerves.

Anxieties about spillage and smell can be considerable. Hence it is not surprising that some colostomates may avoid any social contacts and that 18 per cent refuse to spend a single night away from home (Eardley et al., 1976). Their worries appear closely related to problems in managing the stoma.

Even allowing for the age of many colostomates and progression of the cancer, a substantial proportion have difficulty coping with work.

Preliminary studies of patients after surgery which also results in the loss of key functions, for example, laryngectomy, and urinary diversions suggest that a similar range of problems may occur.

IMPACT OF CHILDHOOD LEUKAEMIA

Leukaemia in a child poses a serious stress for any family. A major problem concerns whether the child will prove to be a survivor or not. Recent studies have shown that all the family can be affected adversely. The parents may become very depressed or anxious (McCarthy, 1975; Kaplan et al., 1973) while up to

50 per cent of the children may develop behavioural problems such as school refusal, attacks of unexplained abdominal pain, wetting the bed and temper tantrums (Howarth, 1972).

As in the case of patients after mastectomy and colostomy few parents mention their problems to anyone in a position to help.

Provision of Counselling

While further studies are needed to clarify the extent and nature of the psychological problems associated with specific cancers it is already clear that much could be done to reduce or prevent them.

Some centres are trying to achieve this by the provision of counselling before and after surgery or after diagnosis when medical treatments are used. The scheme used in the Memorial Hospital, New York for women undergoing mastectomy is a good example of this approach (Dietz, 1969).

Each woman is seen preoperatively by the surgeon who provides detailed information about the possible procedures they may have to undergo. After surgery they are seen both individually and in a group by the nurse, physiotherapist and social worker. The aim of the daily group meetings is to allow the women to be given advice about the exercises which they should carry out, breast prostheses, and an opportunity to discuss among themselves the fears and worries they have about how they will cope when they return home. Particular emphasis is placed on the team approach and the physiotherapist is encouraged to play a key part (Schmid, 1974). A couples' group is also held to which husbands are invited.

Their team approach contrasts with the use of specially trained nurses (Maguire, 1976) who see the women individually before and after surgery, provide advice and support, monitor their subsequent progress and give feedback to both the hospital and community care teams. The effectiveness of such liaison nurses in reducing the emotional problems after mastectomy has yet to be evaluated. However, early experience of their use in a scheme at the University Hospital of South Manchester suggests that they may prove very valuable. It has been claimed that such specially trained nurses have a particularly valuable part to play as stoma therapists after colostomy (Saunders, 1976) or in leukaemia clinics (Foley and McCarthy, 1976).

Both the team and liaison nurse approaches may enlist the aids of volunteers who themselves have undergone but recovered well from the particular treatment, for example colostomy, mastectomy, or laryngectomy. Such volunteers are usually provided by the relevant patient association. These volunteers have the great advantage of having been through the experience themselves and can provide visible evidence that it is possible to survive and still look very attractive. Despite this, many doctors object to their use on the grounds that they may have neurotic reasons for helping others or may die. However, careful selection and training of these volunteers can do much to overcome these objections (Markels, 1973).

The Role of the Physiotherapist

One of the main difficulties in trying to help patients with cancer is their reluctance to disclose how worried they are. Only a third of those who develop emotional problems will discuss them with someone who is in a position to help. The situation is made worse by the failure of most of the staff to ask how the patient is faring emotionally.

It is, therefore, most important that those staff who come into close contact with the patient are alert to any signs of distress and if they notice these, are prepared to ask why the patient is distressed. This will usually lead the patients to mention their real worries and allow the physiotherapist to decide whether she can provide the necessary reassurance or should report the matter to the medical and nursing staff.

Even when there are no obvious signs of distress the physiotherapist should make a general enquiry as to how the patient is feeling, not physically, but in his or her spirits. This will usually reveal that the patient is much more anxious or depressed than she appears to be on the surface.

The emphasis on early ambulation after surgery means that the physiotherapist sees a lot of the patient in the immediate postoperative period. She is thus, well placed to note any evidence that the patient is unduly upset by the scar, colostomy or complications such as swelling. Where she finds the patient will not look at the wound or appliance she should gently enquire as to the reasons for this avoidance. She should then encourage the patient to look at the specific area and reassure him that it will all settle down, and deal with any other worries the patient expresses about it.

The encouragement of self-care activities is particularly important in reducing the risk of 'invalidism' and increasing self-confidence. Hence exercises to restore arm movement after mastectomy which allow the women to comb their hair and apply lipstick can be of great value in overcoming fears of 'looking repulsive'.

In recurrent and advanced disease the physiotherapist may also play a crucial role in helping patients make the best of their disabilities. From a psychological viewpoint it is important that the physical goals set are carefully planned, realistic, and will lead to an improvement in the quality of the patient's life. When the patient appears resistive to physiotherapy the possibility of depression, anxiety, other psychological problems or difficulties at home should be considered.

ANSWERING DIFFICULT QUESTIONS

One reason why many of those who are concerned with cancer patients avoid asking about their feelings, is the fear that they may be asked questions about the cancer and its prognosis which they are unsure how to answer. The physiotherapist's uncertainty may be due to the fact that it is often seen as the doctor's job to decide what patients should be told. She may, therefore, feel she cannot divulge any information. It may also stem from her realistic awareness that very little is yet known about the psychological effects of telling versus not-telling (McIntosh 1974; McIntosh 1976).

It will, therefore, be important that she first finds out from the medical, surgical or radiotherapy team what their policy is for each patient. Where this has not been discussed or decided, her question may provoke them to do so. Otherwise there is a risk that the patient may be given different information by different people. This inconsistency can lead to much emotional distress and suspicion of the true diagnosis. For similar reasons lies should be avoided. The physiotherapist who is prepared to reflect the difficult question back by saying 'why do you ask' may find the patient provides a clear indication of what she already knows or talks in a way that suggests she does not want to know the nature of her illness.

The practice of telling the husband or close family, but not the woman is fairly common, especially when the disease is advanced. While it has been claimed that this 'collusion' protects the patient, it seems more likely that it puts both partners under a terrible strain.

THE WOMAN WHO FAILS TO COPE

When a patient becomes especially anxious, depressed, complains of sexual problems, and there is a discrepancy between her good physical recovery and her inability to cope at home, consideration should be given to psychological help. While it is not yet certain what the exact merits of psychotropic drugs versus counselling are at the moment, the following guidelines can be given.

CONTINUED MOOD DISTURBANCE

The patient who complains that she has felt very lowspirited for some weeks to an extent that it is much greater than usual, has been so low as to wonder if life is worth living, has had difficulty in coping with her chores will usually benefit from the opportunity to talk about her feelings and from a tricyclic antidepressant drug such as Tryptizol (amitriptyline).

When the complaints are of feeling very tense, on edge, palpitations, sweating or headaches, anxiety relieving drugs, for example Valium (diazepam), may be tried.

SEXUAL PROBLEMS

When a patient mentions that he no longer gets enjoyment from sex but expresses a wish to have help he and his partner might benefit from an approach developed by Masters and Johnson (Bancroft 1975). However, we do not yet know just how much these sexual problems of patients after treatment for cancer could be helped by this kind of approach and research is needed to evaluate this.

EMOTIONAL SURVIVAL

Working with cancer patients can be a harrowing experience, especially when the patients with whom the physiotherapist has built up a good relationship fare badly and die. It is important that staff acknowledge how they are affected and have an opportunity of sharing their feelings with colleagues in a supportive atmosphere such as a staff group.

Acknowledgements

This chapter would not have been possible without the generous support of the Cancer Research Campaign.

References

1. Bancroft, J. (1975). 'The Behavioural approach to marital problems', *British Journal of Medical Psychology*, **48**, 147.
2. Chesser, E. S. and Anderson, J. L. (1975). 'Treatment of Breast Cancer: Doctor/Patient Communications and Psychosocial Implications', *Proceedings of the Royal Society of Medicine*, **68**, 793.
3. Devlin, B. H., Plant, J. A. and Griffin, M. (1971). 'Aftermath of surgery for anorectal cancer', *British Medical Journal*, **3**, 413.
4. Dietz, J. H. (1969). 'Rehabilitation of the Cancer Patient', *Medical Clinics of North America*, **53**, 607.
5. Downie, P. A. (1976). 'Post-mastectomy survey', *Nursing Mirror*, March, **25**, 65.

6. Eardley, A., George, D., Davis F., Schofield, P., Wilson, M., Wakefield, J. and Sellwood, R. A. (1976). 'Colostomy: the consequences of surgery', *Clinical Oncology*, **2**, 277.
7. Foley, G. V. and McCarthy, A. M. (1976). 'The child with leukaemia in a special haematology clinic', *American Journal of Nursing*, **76**, 1115.
8. Greer, S. (1976). *Personal Communication*.
9. Holland, J. C. (1973). *Psychological aspects of cancer in Cancer Medicine*, Eds. J. F. Holland and E. Frei. Philadelphia: Lea & Febiger.
10. Howarth, R. V. (1972). 'The psychiatry of terminal illness in children', *Proceedings of the Royal Society of Medicine*, **65**, 1039.
11. Kaplan, D. M., Grobstein, R., and Smith, A. (1976). 'Measuring and predicting the impact of severe illness in families. Health and Social Work.' To be published.
12. Knopf, A. (1974). *Cancer: Changes in opinion after 7 years of public education in Lancaster*, Manchester Regional Committee on Cancer.
13. Maguire, G. P. (1976). 'The psychological and social sequelae of mastectomy', *Modern Perspectives in Psychiatric Aspects of Surgery*, Ed. J. Howells. New York: Bruner-Mazel.
14. Markels, W. M. (1971). 'The American cancer society's programme for the rehabilitation of the breast cancer patient', *Cancer*, **28**, 1676.
15. McCarthy, M. (1975). 'Psychiatric symptoms in mothers of children with leukaemia.' To be published.
16. McIntosh, J. (1974). Processes of communication, information seeking and control associated with cancer: a selective review of the literature', *Social Science and Medicine*, **8**, 167.
17. McIntosh, J. (1976). 'Patient awareness and desire for information about diagnosed but undisclosed malignant disease', *Lancet*, **ii**, 300.
18. Saunders, B. (1976). 'Clinical nurse consultant in stoma care', *Nursing Mirror*, May, **13**, 54.
19. Schmid, W. L., Kiss, M. and Hibert, L. (1974). 'The team approach to rehabilitation after mastectomy', *Journal of the Association of Operating Room Nurses*, **19**, 821.
20. Williams, E. M., Cruikshank, A. and Walker, W. M. (1972). *Public opinion on cancer: a survey of attitudes in South East Wales*, Tenovus Information Centre, Cardiff.

Glossary

ablation The removal of a part by surgery, drugs or radioactive means
adenocarcinoma A tumour arising in glandular tissue
astrocytoma A glioma, usually found in the cerebral hemispheres of an adult or cerebellum of a child
benign tumour Non-malignant or innocent tumour
betatron An accelerator for electrons which produces a high energy electron beam
biopsy Microscopic examination of tissue taken from the body
cancer or **carcinoma** A malignant tumour
carcinogen A substance which can induce cancer
carcinogenesis The process by which a carcinogen converts normal cells to cancer cells
chondrosarcoma A sarcoma which arises from cartilaginous cells
choriocarcinoma A highly malignant and comparatively rare cancer of the placental tissue
colostomy The formation of an artificial anus, either temporary or permanent, by making an opening into the colon, from the skin
cytology The study of the formation and function of cells
cytotoxic Acting to disorganize the cellular metabolism, e.g. cytotoxic drugs
differentiated A term used in the histological description of tumours, indicating that the cells are so ordered that the tissue of origin can be recognized. They are more likely to indicate a slow-growing tumour
ependymoma A tumour which arises from the lining cells of

the ventricles or the central canal of the spinal cord. They are fairly slow growing

familial polyposis Small projecting masses of tissue occurring in the lower part of the small intestine and colon in members of the same family

histology The science of tissue structure

Hodgkin's disease A disease marked by chronic enlargement of lymph nodes, together with enlargement of the spleen

isotope Each element always has the same number of protons in the nuclei of its atoms but may have different numbers of neutrons. The variations of a particular element with different numbers of neutrons are called different isotopes of that element. E.g. *ordinary hydrogen* has one proton in its nucleus; *heavy hydrogen or deuterium* has one proton and one neutron; *radioactive hydrogen or tritium* has one proton and two neutrons. Thus there are three isotopes which are all hydrogen and will behave chemically as such

leukaemia A disease characterized by the presence of immature leucocytes in the blood

linear accelerator A machine for accelerating sub-atomic particles

liposarcoma A sarcoma arising in fat tissue

mammography The examination of the breast by X-rays

medulloblastoma Classified as a glioma, which is found in children and is attached to the roof of the fourth ventricle

metastasis Spread of the primary tumour to another site

neuroblastoma A malignant tumour arising from the nerve cells of embryonic type

obturator From the Latin *obturare*, to close. That which closes or blocks an opening

osteosarcoma A highly malignant tumour of bone

palliation The achievement of temporary relief

radioisotope Short for radioactive isotope. Most naturally occurring isotopes are stable, i.e. they retain their properties for ever. Some are unstable, i.e. they have nuclei which undergo a process of readjustment and therefore change into isotopes of other elements, and in so doing they emit ionising radiation. It is now possible to convert stable isotopes into unstable ones thus creating radioactive forms of all elements

remission No evidence of the disease after all known physical and laboratory examination

retinoblastoma A congenital and frequently hereditary tumour arising from the retina of the embryo

rodent ulcer A slow-growing and potentially invasive tumour involving soft tissue and bone, often a basal cell carcinoma

sarcoma A malignant tumour arising from embryonic connective tissue

undifferentiated A term used in the histological description of tumours indicating that the cells are utterly disorganized so that the tissue of origin cannot be defined. They are usually rapidly growing and highly malignant and are sometimes called anaplastic

References

Atkins, Hedley, Hayward, J. L., Klugman, D. J. & Wayte, A. B. (1972). 'Treatment of Early Breast Cancer: A Report after Ten Years of a Clinical Trial', *British Medical Journal*, 2, 423.

Bagshawe, K. D. (1972). 'Developments of New Anti-Cancer Drugs', included in *Cancer at the Crossroads and the Challenge for the Future*, p. 23. Ed. Ronald W. Raven. William Heinemann Medical Books Ltd.

Balmforth, J. (1958). 'The Development and Scope of Cytology in the Diagnosis of Malignancy', *Medical Press*, **CCXXXX**, 665.

Barlow, Donald (1969). 'A Cough-Belt to Prevent and Treat Postoperative Pulmonary Complications', *Lancet*, 2, 736.

Burkitt, D. P. (1972). 'Cancer of the Colon and Rectum, Epidemiology and Suggested Causative Factors', Walker Prize Lecture included in *Cancer at the Crossroads and the Challenge for the Future*, p. 103. Ed. Ronald W. Raven. William Heinemann Medical Books Ltd.

Cartwright, Frederick F. (1972). *Disease and History*. Hart Davis, London.

Cook, H. Peter (1971). 'Prostheses after Major Surgery of the Head and Neck', included in *Symposium on the Rehabilitation of the Cancer Disabled*, p. 58. Ed. Ronald W. Raven. William Heinemann Medical Books Ltd.

Cyriax, James H. (1971). *A Textbook of Orthopaedic Medicine*, Vols. 1 and 2. Baillière Tindall, London.

Downie, Patricia A. (1971). 'The Physiotherapist and the Patient with Cancer'. *Physiotherapy*, 57, 117.

Downie, P. A. (1973). 'Physiotherapy and the Care of the Progressively Ill Patient', 1. The Role of the Physiotherapist,

Nursing Times, **69**, 892; 2. The Unconscious and Bedridden Patient, *Nursing Times*, **69**, 922; 3. Physiotherapy for the Paralysed Patient, *Nursing Times*, **69**, 958.

Downie, Patricia A. (1974). 'The Patient with a Cancerous Disease', *Queen's Nursing Journal*, **16**, 254.

Gillbe, P. (1973). 'Xeroradiography of the Breast', *Radiography*, **XXXIX**, No. 461, 127.

Gillis, Leon (1959). 'Prosthetic Replacement in Cases of Cancer', Ch. 14 included in *Cancer*, Vol 6, p. 347. Ed. Ronald W. Raven. Butterworth & Co. Ltd.

Guardini, Romano (1954). *The Last Things*. Burns & Oates, London.

Haenszel, W. & Kurihara, M. (1968). 'Study of Japanese Migrants. I. Mortality from cancer and other diseases among Japanese in the United States', *Journal of the National Cancer Institute*, **40**, 43.

Harrison, D. F. M. (1973). 'Laryngeal carcinoma', *British Journal of Hospital Medicine*, November, 597.

Hawker, Margaret (1974). *Geriatrics for Physiotherapists and the Allied Professions*, p. 60. Faber & Faber.

Holt, J. A. G. (1973). 'Thermography in Screening', *Health and Social Services Journal*, February, 305.

Leaflet of Advice for Patients following Mastectomy (1971). The Marie Curie Memorial Foundation, London.

Markham, M. M. (1970). 'The Relief of Pain', *Nursing Times*, 10 December, p. 1579.

Physiotherapy Helps Nursing (1962). Nursing Times Publication, Macmillan & Co. Ltd., London.

Raven, R. W. (1973). Address at the first meeting of the British Association of Surgical Oncology, included in *Ann. Roy. Coll. Surg. Engl.*, 53.

Rendle Short, A. (1953). *The Bible and Modern Medicine*. Paternoster Press.

Robbie, D. S. (1969). 'Management of Intractable Pain in Advanced Cancer of the Rectum', *Proc. Roy. Soc. Med.*, **63**, 115.

Robbie, D. S. (1971). 'Abolition of Pain', included in *Symposium on the Rehabilitation of the Cancer Disabled*, p. 26. Ed. Ronald W. Raven. William Heinemann Medical Books Ltd.

Roe, F. J. C. (1971). 'Prevention of Cancer', *Physiotherapy*, 57, 109.

Scott, Ronald Bodley (1970). 'Cancer Chemotherapy. The First Twenty-five Years', *British Medical Journal*, 4, 259.

Shedd, D., Bakamjian, V., Sako, K., Mann, M., Barba, S. & Scharf, N. (1972). 'Reed-Fistula Method of Speech Rehabilitation after Laryngectomy', *American Journal of Surgery*, 124, 510.

Simons, Bernard C., Lehman, Justus F., Taylor, Neal & Delateur, Barbara J. (1968). 'Prosthetic Management of Hemicorporectomy', *Orthotics and Prosthetics*, June, p. 63.

Simpson, J. D. (1974). 'Nuclear Medicine', *Nursing Times*, 15 August, 1260.

Sister Magdalen (1974). 'Lumen Christi', *The Way of Life*, 6, 148.

Tait, Vera (1971). 'Restoration of Function following Laryngectomy, including Electronic Aids', included in *Symposium on the Rehabilitation of the Cancer Disabled*, p. 75. Ed. Ronald W. Raven. William Heinemann Medical Books Ltd.

Thomas, Betty J. (1974). 'Coping with the devastation of head and neck cancer', *RN Magazine*, 37, 10, 25.

Wallace, David M. (1972). 'Solution of Problems caused by Colostomy and Ileal Conduits', included in *Symposium on the Rehabilitation of the Cancer Disabled*, p. 87. Ed. Ronald W. Raven. William Heinemann Medical Books Ltd.

Watson-Jones, R. (1952). *Fractures and Joint Injuries*, Vol. II, 1021. Churchill Livingstone.

Williams, H. A. (1972). *True Resurrection*, p. 142. Mitchell Beazley, London.

Wolfe, J. N., Dooley, R. P. & Hawkins, L. E. (1971). 'Xeroradiography of the breast. A Comparative study with conventional film mammography', *Cancer*, 28, 1569.

Zirkle, Thomas J. & Thompson, Ralph J. (1974). 'Repairing the face and neck after radical excision', *RN Magazine*, 37, 10.

Bibliography

Bagshawe, K. D. (Ed. 1975). *Medical Oncology. Medical aspects of malignant disease*, Blackwell Scientific Publications.

Bromley, Ida (1976). *Tetraplegia and Paraplegia. A Guide for Physiotherapists*, Churchill Livingstone.

Cash, Joan (Ed. 1974). *Neurology for Physiotherapists*, Faber & Faber.

Cash, Joan E. (Ed. 1975). *Chest, Heart and Vascular Disorders for Physiotherapists*, Faber & Faber.

Deeley, T. J., Fish, E. J., & Gough, M. A. (1974). *A Guide to Oncological Nursing*, Churchill Livingstone.

Ellison Nash, D. F. (1973). *The Principles and Practice of Surgery for Nurses and Allied Professions*, Edward Arnold.

Gaskell, D. V. & Webber, B. A. (1977). *The Brompton Hospital Guide to Chest Physiotherapy*, Blackwell Scientific Publications.

Harris, R. J. C. (Ed. 1970). *What We Know About Cancer*, George Allen & Unwin Ltd.

Healey, John E. (Ed. 1970). *Ecology of the Cancer Patient*, The Interdisciplinary Communications Associates Inc., Washington D.C.

Hinton, John (1968). *Dying*, Penguin Books.

Humm, W. (1965). *Rehabilitation of the Lower Limb Amputee*, Baillière Tindall.

Lack, S. & Lamerton, R. (Joint Eds. 1974). *The Hour of Our Death* (a record of a conference on the Care of the Dying), Geoffrey Chapman, London.

Lamerton, R. (1974). *Care of the Dying*, Priory Press.

Raven, Ronald W. & Roe, F. J. C. (Joint Eds. 1970). *The Prevention of Cancer*, Butterworth & Co. Ltd.

Stell, P. M. & Maran, A. G. D. (1972). *Head and Neck Surgery*, William Heinemann Medical Books Ltd.

Taylor, Selwyn & Cotton, Leonard (1973). *A Short Textbook of Surgery*, The English Universities Press Ltd.

Tiffany, Robert (Ed. 1978) *Oncology for Nurses and Health Care Professionals*, in two volumes, George Allen & Unwin.

TNM Classification of Malignant Tumours, UICC, Geneva.

Walter, J. (1971). *Cancer and Radiotherapy*, Churchill Livingstone.

Wilkinson, James (1973). *The Conquest of Cancer*, Hart-Davis MacGibbon.

Useful organizations

The Colostomy Welfare Group, 38–9 Eccleston Square, London S.W.1.
The Ileostomy Association, Drove Cottage, Kempshott, Basingstoke, Hants.
The Leukaemia Research Fund, 61 Great Ormond Street, London WC1N 3JJ.
The Malcolm Sargent Cancer Fund for Children, 56 Redcliffe Square, London S.W.5.
The Marie Curie Memorial Foundation, 124 Sloane Street, London SW1X 9BP.
The Mastectomy Association, 1 Colworth Road, Croydon, Surrey.
The National Association of Laryngectomy Clubs, c/o Hon. Sec. Mr. T. Bradley, 7 Forest Lodge, Dartmouth Road, London S.E.23.
The National Society for Cancer Relief, Michael Sobell House, 30 Dorset Square, London N.W.1.
The Women's National Cancer Control Campaign, 44 Russell Square, London W.C.1.
The Cancer Research Campaign, 2 Carlton House Terrace, London SW1Y 5AR.
The Imperial Cancer Research Fund, Lincoln's Inn Fields, London WC2A 3PX.
The Cancer Information Association, Gloucester Green, Oxford.
The Manchester Regional Committee on Cancer, Kinnaird Road, Manchester.
The Merseyside Cancer Education Committee, 8 Victoria Street, Liverpool.

Homes and hospices

St. Christopher's Hospice, Lawrie Park Road, London SE26 6DZ.
The Hostel of God, 29 North Side, Clapham Common, London S.W.4.
St. Joseph's Hospice, Mare Street, London E.8.
St. Barnabas Home, Columbia Drive, Worthing, Sussex, BN13 2QF.
The Douglas Macmillan House, Christchurch, Hampshire.
St. Luke's Nursing Home, Sheffield.
St. Ann's Hospice, Cheadle Hulme, Manchester.
The Douglas Macmillan Home, Stoke on Trent, Staffordshire.
The Cynthia Spencer Home, The Manfield Hospital, Northampton.
Sir Michael Sobell Home, The Churchill Hospital, Oxford.

THE MARIE CURIE MEMORIAL FOUNDATION HOMES

Edenhall, Hampstead, London N.W.3.
Tidcombe Hall, Tiverton, Devon.
Hunter's Hill, Glasgow
Fairmile, Edinburgh.
Sunnybank, Liverpool.
Conrad House, Newcastle upon Tyne.
Arden Lea, Ilkley, Yorkshire.
Harestone Nursing Home, Caterham, Surrey.
Holme Tower, Penarth, Glamorgan.
Warren Pearl Nursing Home, Solihull, Warwickshire.
Beaconfield, Belfast.

ADDITIONAL HOMES AND HOSPICES ARE UNDER CONSTRUCTION OR BEING PLANNED AT:

Milton Keynes, Bucks; Birmingham; Newcastle upon Tyne; Norwich; Nottingham; Edinburgh.

RECENTLY OPENED HOMES:

Michael Sobell House, Mount Vernon Hospital, Northwood, Middlesex.
Countess Mountbatten House, Moorgreen Hospital, Southampton, Hampshire.
Roxburgh House, Royal Victoria Hospital, Dundee.
Roxburgh House, Tor-na-Dee Hospital, Aberdeen.

Useful addresses of cancer organizations and special homes in the United States of America and Canada

The American Cancer Society.
National Headquarters
777 Third Avenue, New York. N.Y. 10017
Divisional Offices are to be found in most states; addresses are located in Yellow Pages.
The American Cancer Society is a voluntary organization and nationally organized to fight cancer through balanced programmes of research, education and patient service and rehabilitation. There are five specific departments: Public Education, Professional Education, Service and Rehabilitation, and Research.

International Association of Laryngectomees
National Office
777 Third Avenue, New York, N.Y. 10017
Sponsored by the American Cancer Society.
Coordinates 'Lost Chord' clubs, and by 1975 had 228 affiliated clubs in 44 states and 11 foreign countries.

Reach to Recovery (Mastectomy Rehabilitation Programme)
National Office
777 Third Avenue, New York, N.Y. 10017
Sponsored by the American Cancer Society with organized groups in all the Divisions. Addresses to be found in local Yellow Pages.

HOSPITALS AND HOMES FOR PATIENTS WITH ADVANCED CANCER

The Calvary Hospital, McCoombs Road, Bronx, New York 10452.
Hospice Inc, Prospect Street, New Haven, Connecticut 06511.
(At present this unit only runs a Home Care Service; a Hospice is planned).
St. Monica's Home, Roxbury, Boston, Massachusetts.

The Canadian Cancer Society.
National Headquarters
25 Adelaide Street East, Toronto, Ontario M5C 1Y2
Divisional Offices are to be found in all Provinces; their addresses are located in Yellow Pages.
Like the American Cancer Society they sponsor Reach to Recovery and Lost Chord Clubs (part of the International Association of Laryngectomees)

Special Units for the Care of Dying Patients
Palliative Care Unit, The Royal Victoria Hospital, Montreal, Quebec.
Extended Care Unit, St. Boniface Hospital, Winnipeg, Manitoba.

Index

Ablation of ductless glands, 39, 86, 90
Adrenalectomy, 39, 87
   physiotherapy following, 87 et seq.
Amputation,
   above and below knee, 124
   disarticulation of hip, 51, 123
   hemi-pelvectomy, 123
   role of the physiotherapist following, 123
Anaemia, 155, 158
Angiography, 33
Ankylosing spondylitis, 24
Anorexia, 152, 156, 160
Apocrypha, 22

Backache, 130
Biopsy,
   definition, 34
   frozen technique, 34
   methods of taking, 34
Bladder cancer, 112, 131
   physiotherapy in, 113
   surgery in, 113, 114
Bone tumours, 122
   physiotherapy in, 123
   prognosis of, 124
   secondary, 125
   types, 122
Brain tumours, *see* cerebral tumours

Breast cancer,
   fear of, 80
   lymphoedema in, 92
   psychological impact of, 174–84
   treatment of advanced, 86, 90
   types of operation for, 80
   see also mastectomy

Cachexia, 160
Cancer,
   astronomical associations, 21
   biblical references to, 22
   causation, 23
   definition, 15
   environmental factors, 24
   historical associations, 21–23
   planning of medical treatment, 35
   predisposing factors of, 25
   prevention and control of, 26
   supersitions about, 23
Cancer education, 26
   role of the physiotherapist in, 147 et seq.
Carcinogens, 23
Case-histories, 51, 60, 63, 67, 72, 75, 87, 107, 118, 142
Cautery, 22
Cerebral tumours, 72, 115
   disability from, 116
   radiotherapy for, 79, 116
   rehabilitation for, 78, 117

INDEX

Cerebral tumours—*cont.*
  surgery for, 116
  types of, 115
Cervical node block dissection, 98
Chemotherapy, 42–4, 56
  definition, 42, 56
  infusion, 61
  nutritional problems following, 157
  perfusion, 61
  principles of physiotherapy in, 57
  precautions, for physiotherapy following, 135
  rehabilitation, 59 *et seq.*
  side-effects, 43
  systemic, 56
Colon cancer,
  colostomy after, 182
  predisposing factors, 25
  surgery for, 38
Colostomy, psychological impact following, 182
Cough belt, 112
Counselling for patients with cancer, 183
Cytology, 34

Death, philosophy of approach to, 136
Diagnosis of cancer,
  clinical, 30
  impact of, 174
  special facilities for, 31 *et seq.*
Diets, 161
Dying, care of the, 136
  physiotherapy for, 74, 137

Ependymoma, rehabilitation after, 75 *et seq.*
Euthanasia, 139

Frenkel's exercises, 60, 76, 145

Halsted radical mastectomy, 37, 80
Head and neck tumours,
  physiotherapy in, 48, 96 *et seq.*
  radiotherapy for, 40
  rehabilitation following, 106
  surgery for, 38, 99, *et seq.*
  see also jaw surgery, laryngectomy
Hemi-mandibulectomy, 102
  physiotherapy following, 102–5
  reconstructive surgery following, 103
Herodotus, 22
Herpes zoster, 24
Hippocrates, 25
Hodgkin's disease, 41, 67, 117
Hypophysectomy, 39, 90

Immunotherapy, 44
Isotopes, 40
  scanning by, 33
  half life of, 33

Jaw surgery, 101
  hemi-mandibulectomy, 102
  physiotherapy following, 104
  rehabilitation after, 106
Jobst compression unit, 93

Laminectomy, 67, 117
Laryngectomy and pharyngo-laryngo-oesophagectomy, 99–101
  physiotherapy following, 100
  rehabilitation following, 100–1
  Swallow Clubs for, 100
Leukaemia, 42, 56, 60
Lung cancer, *see* thoracic surgery
Lymphoedema, 92
  treatment of, 92–5
Lymphography, 32

Malabsorption, 154, 158, 162

Mammography, 31
Mastectomy,
  counselling for patients following, 183
  general rehabilitation following, 85–6
  lymphoedema following, 92
    treatment of, 92–5
  physiotherapy following, 82–5
  prostheses following, 86, 179
  psychological impact following, 174
  types of, 37, 80
Metastases (deposits), 28, 52, 125, 144
  bone, 91
  from breast cancer, 15, 86
  surgery for, 39
Myeloma, 63, 117
  aetiology, 63
  rehabilitation following, 63–5

Napoleon, death of, 22
Nerve blocking, 145
  physiotherapy following, 145
Nutrition and cancer, 152 *et seq.*
  following radiotherapy, 156
  following surgery, 154
  needs following chemotherapy, 157
  psychological problems, 160

Oesophagectomy, 155
Oncology, definition of, 16
Oophorectomy, 36, 86

Pain,
  causes of, 144
  definition, 144
  general aspects of, 146
  nerve blocking for, 39, 145
  role of physiotherapist in treatment of, 145
  surgical relief of, 39, 145

Pancreas, surgery for cancer of, 38
Paraplegia due to spinal compression,
  physiotherapy and rehabilitation for, 67 *et seq.*, 117 *et seq.*
Parenteral feeding, 163
Pathological fracture, 39, 52, 125
Patey mastectomy, 37, 81
  physiotherapy following, 82
Paul of Aegina, 21
Physiotherapy,
  development of, 11–12
  following chemotherapy, 56 *et seq.*
  following radiotherapy, 66 *et seq.*
  in the presence of bone metastases, 91
  principles, 111–12
  see also case-histories
Precautions for physiotherapists, 130–5
Psychological impact of cancer,
  general, 172
  counselling for, 183
  following drug treatments, 173
  following radiotherapy, 173
  following surgery, 177
  on the physiotherapist and other staff, 187
  on sexual problems, 187

Radiation monitoring badge, 131
Radiation Protection Act, 26
Radioactive Substances Act, 131
Radiotherapy,
  definition of, 39
  external, 39, 66
  historical background of, 39
  internal, 40, 66
  nutritional problems following, 156
  physiotherapy following 67 *et seq.*

INDEX

Radiotherapy—*cont.*
  precautions for physiotherapy following, 131
  side-effects of, 40, 116, 156, 173
  treatments, 41
Radium implants, 40, 132
Rehabilitation,
  nutritional aspects of, 161
  philosophy of, 46–53, 169
  team approach to, 53–5

Sarcoma of bone, 122
  radiotherapy for, 66
  surgery for, 37, 122
Scinti-scanning, 33
Screening methods, 26, 30–4
Short-wave diathermy, use of, 130, 134
Smoking, 150
Spinal tumours, 117
  physiotherapy following, 117 *et seq.*
  surgical treatment of, 38, 117
  types of, 117
Stomas, 112
  psychological problems following, 182
  role of physiotherapy in, 113
Surgical treatment of cancer, 36, 80, 96, 111
  curative, 36
  historical background of, 36
  nutritional problems following, 154
  palliative, 38
  precautions for physiotherapy treatment following, 135
  principles of physiotherapy in, 111

Symphysis pubis, excision of, 114
Systemic lupus erythematosus, 25, 119

Team approach, 46, 53, 153, 156, 183
Telling the patient, 54, 137, 175, 185
Terminal care, *see* death; dying, care of the
Thermography, 31
Thoracic tumours,
  causation, 24
  primary, 125
  secondary, 128
  surgical treatment of, 125
    physiotherapy following, 126
  terminal care following, 128
TNM classification, 29
Tube feeding, 162
Tumour,
  behaviour of, 27
  classification of, 29
  definition of, 27
  differentiation of, 28
  pathology, 27

Ultraviolet light, 114, 134, 135

Vincristine, 43, 75
Viruses, 24
Vitamin deficiencies, 168
Vulva, carcinoma of, 114

Weight loss, 153, 159
Wheelchairs, provision of, 118
Wigs, provision of, 43, 79

Xerography, 31